"No one is born a great cook, one learns by doing."
— Julia Child

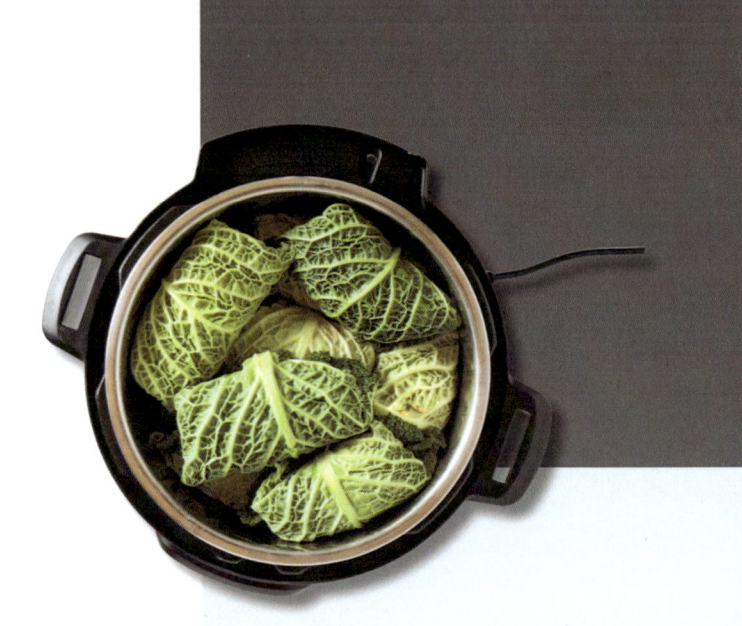

Table of Contents

07   Breakfast

31   Soups & Stews

63   Lunch or Dinner

161   Desserts & Treats

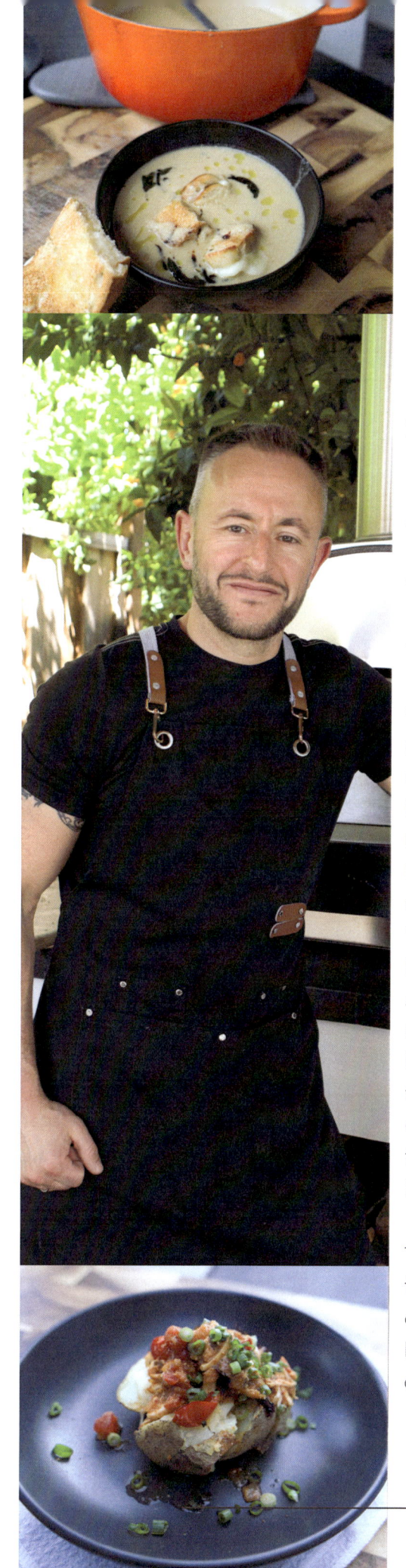

About Me

Hi, I'm Ilya—the guy behind the In the Kitchen with Ilya @inthekitchenwithilya cooking blog. I'm a former tech entrepreneur who now helps people get fit and eat well., with a love for travel, bold flavors, martial arts, and anything that gets the heart rate up.

Now, let's get this out of the way: I'm not a classically trained chef. I don't have 30 years of restaurant experience. I've never yelled "Yes, Chef!" in a commercial kitchen. My background is a little different.

I started my career in the audio-visual and IT space and spent over two decades building a successful business with my brother. Then came 2020—a global reset button we didn't ask for. Like many of you, I suddenly had more time and needed a new outlet to manage the stress. My passion for fitness and travel led me somewhere unexpected: the kitchen.

Back then, I only cooked on weekends for friends and family—grilling steaks, kebabs, and making my signature Georgian comfort dish: Khachapuri. But as I explored global flavors and fitness-friendly ingredients, I started experimenting. And that's how this new chapter began.

Let's be honest: good food is 70% of travel success, and great nutrition is 80% of fitness success. A lot of people think "healthy" and "delicious" can't live on the same plate. In this book, I'll prove that they can—and should.

After every trip, I come back brimming with ideas. But the real challenge? Recreating those flavors at home—fast, healthy, high in protein, and low in empty carbs. So I developed a flexible formula: nutrient-dense, fitness-friendly dishes you can make in around 30 minutes, often using tools like the air fryer, Instant Pot, or waffle maker. (Yes, some recipes take longer—but they're worth it, I promise.)

This book is filled with recipes, time-saving kitchen hacks, fitness tips, and the same nutrition strategies I share with my clients. You don't need a culinary degree to cook from this book. You just need an open mind, a little courage, and a decent spatula.

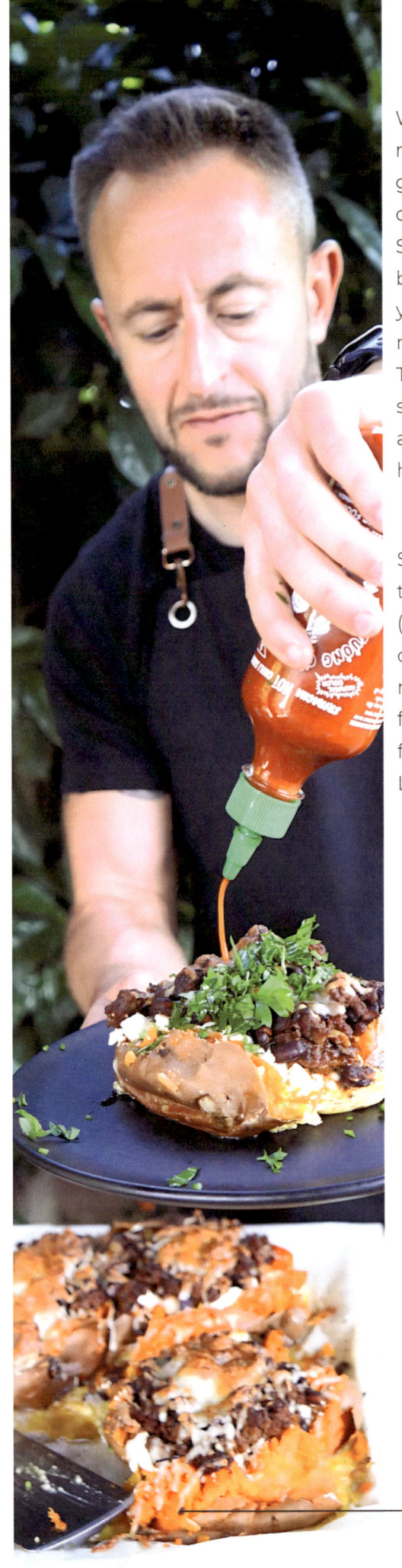

Will you mess up a dish or two? Probably. So what? Most mistakes are fixable—and the wins will be worth it. Once you get a few reps in, you'll be making these meals with your eyes closed.

So why a book in the era of social media overload? Because a book grounds you. It's a trusted companion you can toss on your kitchen counter, get sauce stains on, and flip through for real inspiration—not just another scroll.

This book is for everyday people who want to eat better, cook smarter, and still enjoy the hell out of their food. It's also for anyone who's ever asked, "How can I make something healthy that actually tastes good?"

Special thanks to my wife and kids, who inspire me daily, taste-test my experiments, and offer honest feedback (sometimes too honest). A big shoutout to my brother and his crew, who stop by for post-workout bootcamp meals and never leave hungry. And to my friends at the gym—thank you for always tasting my recipes and giving me honest, no-filter feedback and fresh inspiration.

Let's get cooking!

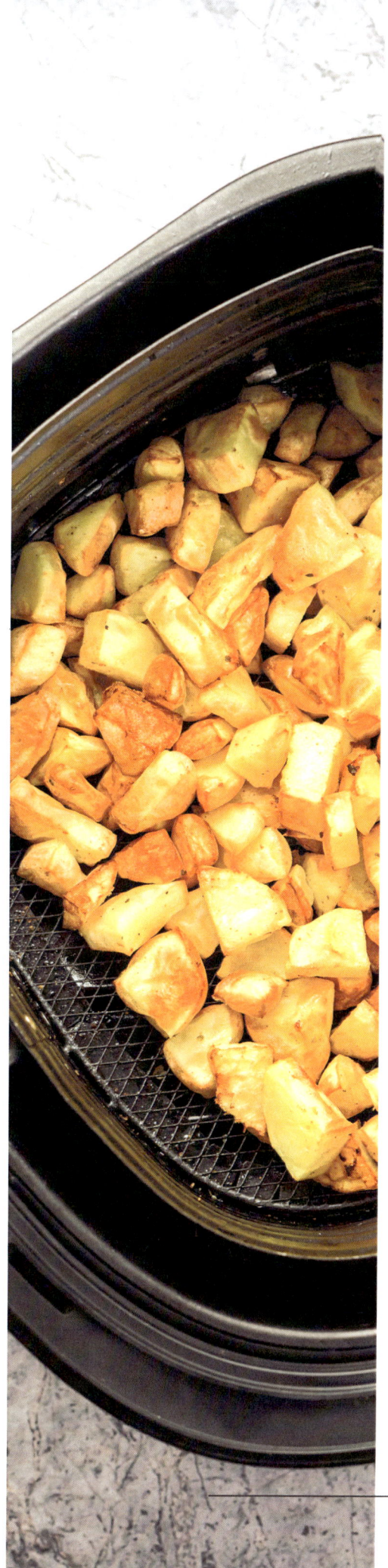

My Go-To Kitchen Sidekicks

No fancy gadgets. Just a couple of modern kitchen tools that pull way more than their weight.

Air Fryer

The air fryer is hands down the hardest-working tool in my kitchen. I've been using mine for over four years, and at this point, I'd rescue it before my blender. It's small, portable, and wildly versatile. Need an oven, fryer, grill, or dehydrator? Done. You can even use it to reheat fries without turning them into sad, soggy potato strips.

I use a 6-quart Cosori model, but any size works—just adjust the batch size and maybe the cooking time a bit. The beauty is in the simplicity.

Why I love it:

- Even cooking – Crisps things up beautifully without burning edges.
- Minimal oil – You get that fried texture with just a spritz of oil.
- Portable & compact – Perfect for keeping the kitchen cool, especially in summer.
- Multipurpose – Use it as an oven, grill, dehydrator, or emergency toaster.
- No preheat drama – Most recipes go straight in, no waiting around.

Instant Pot (Pressure Cooker)

If the air fryer is my right hand, the Instant Pot is my left. For soups, stews, curries, or anything liquid-based, it's a total game-changer. Dump, press, walk away, and come back to a finished meal.

Why I love it:

- One-pot magic – Sauté your aromatics, brown your meat, and cook everything in the same pot.
- Set it and forget it – Great for batch cooking or lazy Sundays.
- Super versatile – From perfectly boiled eggs to tender shredded chicken or even yogurt, it does it all.

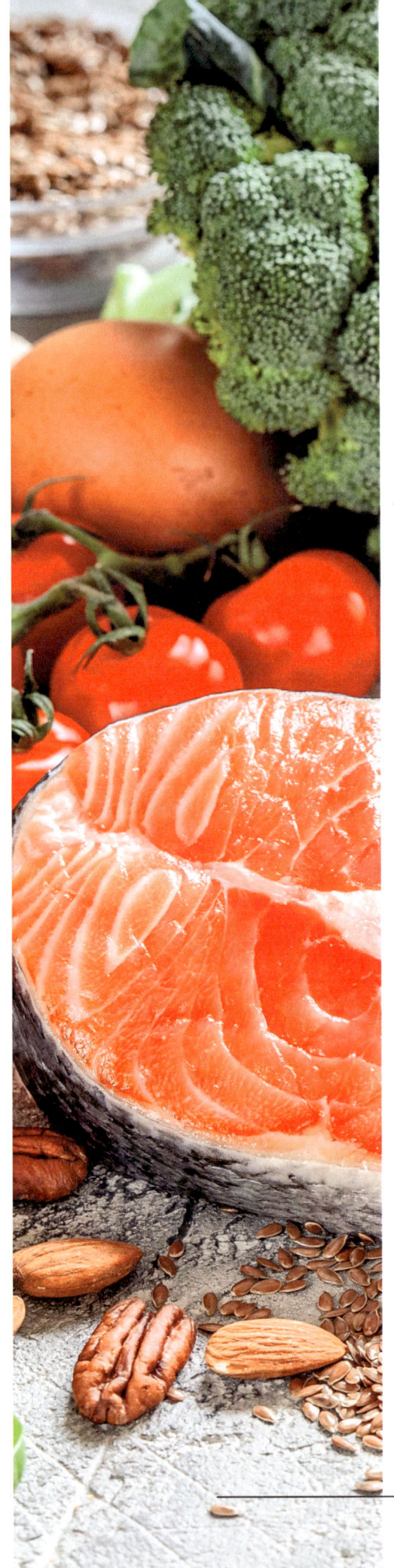

Why High-Protein, Low-Carb Works

Let's clear something up: I'm not anti-carb, and I'm definitely not pushing any trendy diet plans. I don't believe in restrictive eating unless you've got a medical reason and a professional guiding you. What I do believe in? Balanced eating that fuels your body and supports your goals.

The meals in this book follow a simple framework: high in protein, low in sugar and refined carbs, packed with vegetables, and full of flavor. I'm not reinventing the wheel here—I'm just making it spin faster.

So, why protein?

Because whether you're trying to lose weight, build muscle, or just avoid that mid-afternoon energy crash, protein is your best friend. It keeps you full, helps preserve (and build) lean muscle, and boosts your metabolism more than fats or carbs do.

Here's what that looks like in real life:

More animal protein: Think eggs, lean meats, poultry, fish, cottage cheese, and Greek yogurt.

More vegetables: For fiber, fullness, and all the micronutrients your multivitamin wishes it had.

Less sugar and junky fats: Say goodbye to sad pastries and empty-calorie desserts (except the high-protein ones I sneak in here).

And yes, I still eat carbs—I just choose the kind that work with me, not against me. That means complex carbs like sweet potatoes, squash, and legumes when I need fuel, not a crash.

How Much Protein Do You Actually Need?

It depends on your goal, but here's a quick cheat sheet:

Losing fat: 0.7–0.8g per pound
(150 lbs = 105–120g/day)

Maintaining: 0.8–1.0g per pound
(150 lbs = 120–150g/day)

Building muscle: 1.0–1.2g per pound
(150 lbs = 150–180g/day)

Most recipes in this book hit the 30g+ protein mark per serving, which fits perfectly into those targets.

And veggies? Eat them. They're your secret weapon for staying full, keeping your digestion on track, and packing in nutrients.

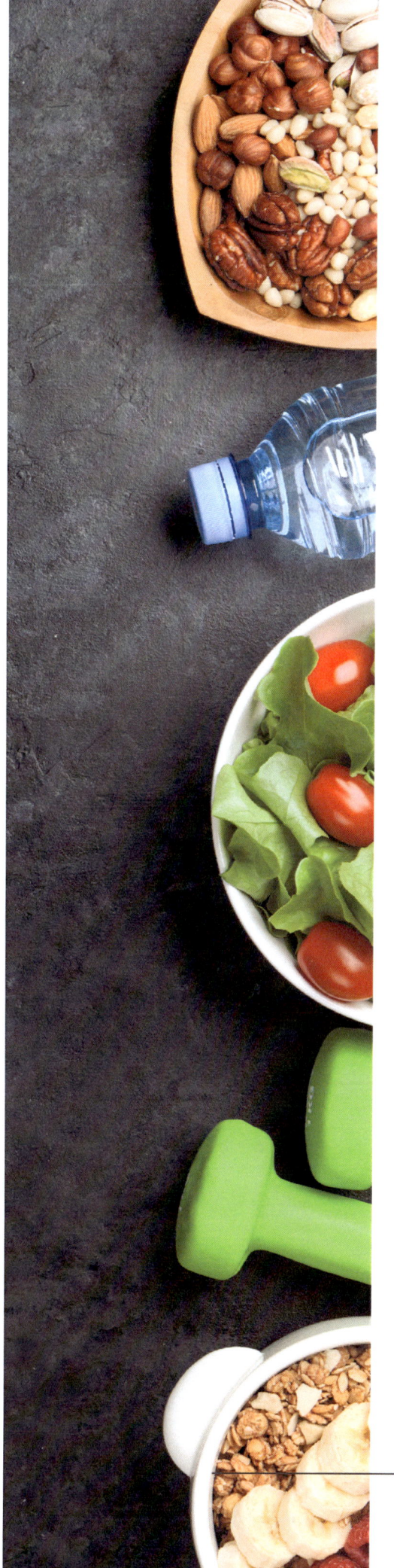

Fitness, Food, and Finding the Time

10,000 steps a day—you've heard it before, and you'll hear it again here. Whether you walk or run them is totally up to you. Pair that with HIIT (high-intensity interval training) a few times a week and strength training at least 3x per week. Why? Because building and maintaining muscle is non-negotiable—especially if you're chasing fat loss, energy, or longevity.

My advice? Make fitness and healthy eating a priority. Once you do that, the time seems to magically appear.

Faster Doesn't Mean Worse

Look—I've got mad respect for traditional cooking. Grandma's lasagna that took 3 hours? Iconic. But here's the truth: if I can make a dish in 30 minutes instead of 90, and it still tastes great, you better believe I'm doing it. That doesn't make the food worse—it just makes it doable. And when something's doable, you're more likely to make it again (instead of reaching for takeout with a side of regret).

This is why I love using modern kitchen tools like the air fryer and Instant Pot. They cut down prep time, simplify steps, and still deliver big on flavor. That's the goal of this book: make healthy cooking faster, not fussier.

QR Codes for Real Help

Every recipe in this book includes a QR code linking to a short video demo. Because let's face it, sometimes watching someone cook it is easier than reading it. Scan, watch, cook.

One Quick Note on Cook Time

Instant Pot recipes do NOT include the time it takes to build pressure. Why? Because it varies. It could take 5 minutes, or it could take 15—depending on how full the pot is and the temperature of your ingredients. So just know: when I say "10 minutes on high pressure," I mean 10 minutes once it gets there.

Disclaimer

I'm not a doctor, registered dietitian, or licensed nutritionist. The advice and recipes in this book are based on personal experience, research, and working with clients who've had real results using these methods. But everyone is different. Please talk to a healthcare provider or dietitian before making big changes to your diet, especially if you have health conditions or specific needs.

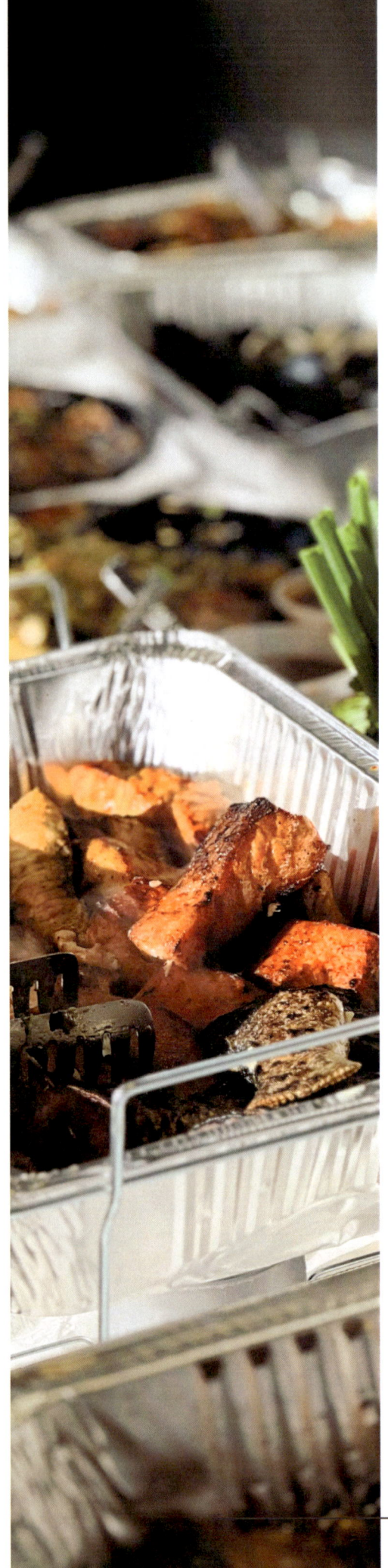

Bonus Section: How to Host a Kickass Party (Without Losing Your Mind)

Straight-up tips from a family that's hosted over 100 of these things. If there's one thing we've learned after a decade of birthdays, game nights, BBQs, and full-blown holiday feasts—it's this: Keep it simple, prep smart, and don't get stuck in the kitchen while everyone else is having a good time. Hosting should feel like fun, not a survival challenge.

1. Use Disposable Cups & Plates
Yes, real dishes look nice. But washing 50 plates the next day? Nope. Grab a stack of solid disposables and move on. Bonus points for compostable ones.

2. Send Invites Early
At least two weeks out. Group chat, text, or an actual invite—doesn't matter. Just don't wing it last minute unless you want a half-empty party and lukewarm hot dogs.

3. Go Individual with Drinks
Skip the punch bowl and gallon jugs. Get cans, bottles, or single-serve cocktails. They stay cold, people grab what they want, and cleanup is a breeze.

4. Set Up the Night Before
Tables, speakers, ice bins—get everything in place the day before. The less you're scrambling on party day, the better. You want to be greeting guests, not hunting for serving spoons.

5. Charcuterie = Appetizer King
No cooking. Just arrange some meats, cheeses, crackers, nuts, maybe olives. Costco has everything you need and nobody's going to complain.

6. Use Your Instant Pot (or Slow Cooker) to Keep Food Warm
No one wants cold rice or room-temp chili. Set your Instant Pot to "Keep Warm" and boom—hot food all night without the hassle.

7. Keep Mains Simple
Roast a salmon, dump rice in the cooker, maybe a one-pot pasta dish. People love good food, not complicated menus. If you're sweating in the kitchen, you're doing it wrong.

8. Let People Bring Stuff
Don't say no when someone offers to help. Just keep it controlled—assign drinks, dessert, or sides. Less work for you, more variety on the table.

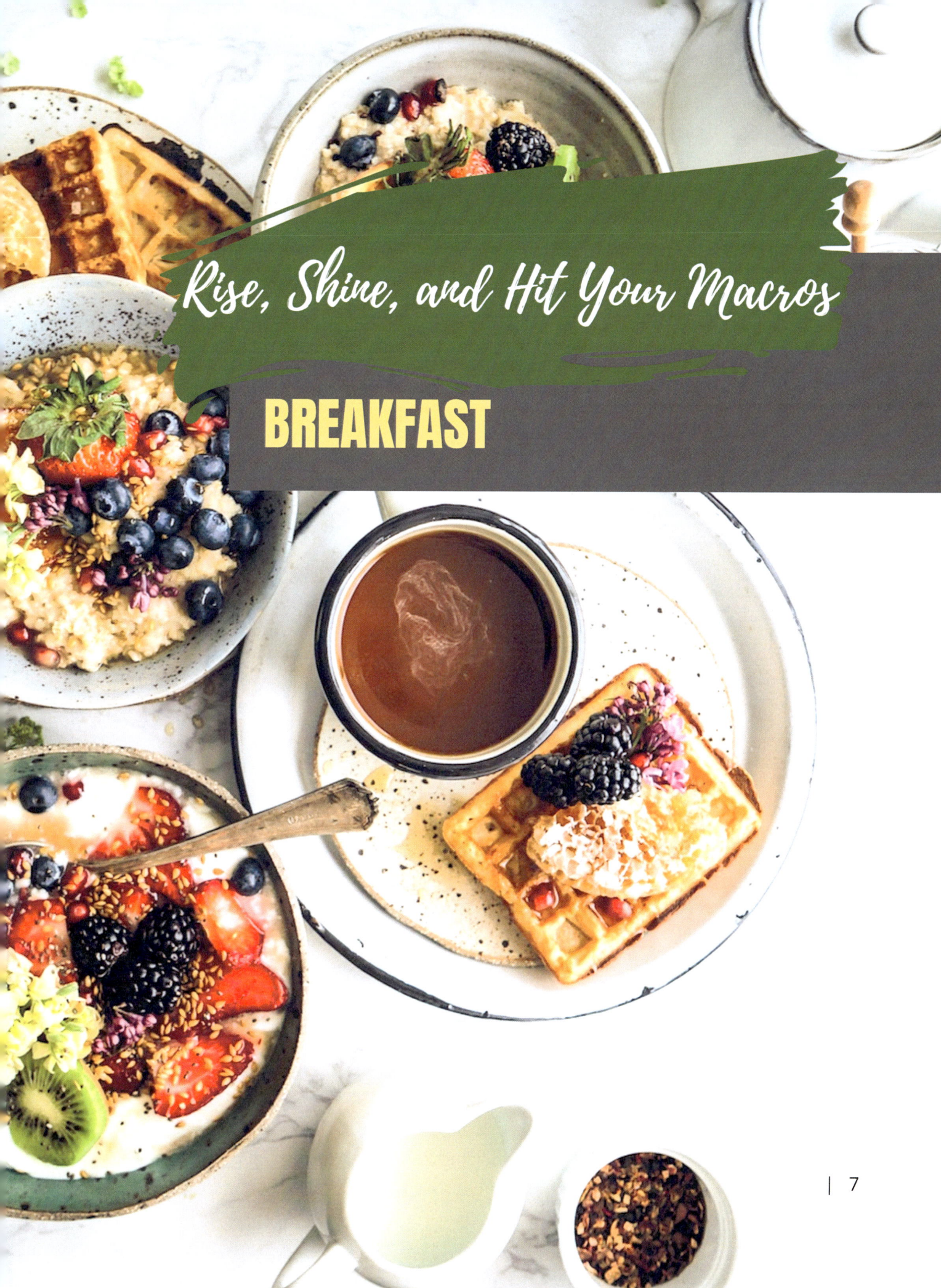

Rise, Shine, and Hit Your Macros

BREAKFAST

PROTEIN-PACKED SHAKSHUKA WITH BEANS AND FETA

Shakshuka: the one-pan wonder that turns simple ingredients into a bold, hearty meal. Originating from North Africa and popular in Israel, it's all about spicy tomato sauce, poached eggs, and now—extra protein with beans and feta.

Ingredients

- 1 tbsp olive oil
- 1 medium onion, chopped
- 1 red bell pepper, chopped
- 3 cloves garlic, minced
- 1 tsp ground cumin
- 1 tsp paprika
- 1/4 tsp chili powder
- 4 fresh tomatoes, diced
- 1 can (15 oz) cooked beans (black, kidney, or chickpeas), drained
- 4 large eggs
- 1/2 cup crumbled feta cheese
- Salt and pepper, to taste
- Fresh cilantro or parsley for garnish
- Naan or crusty bread

Instructions

- Sauté: heat oil in a skillet over medium. Cook onion and bell pepper for 5-7 minutes. Add garlic, cumin, paprika, and chili powder. Cook 1-2 minutes.
- Simmer: stir in tomatoes and beans. Season with salt and pepper. Simmer 10 minutes.
- Eggs: make 4 wells, crack an egg into each. Cover and cook 5-7 minutes, until eggs are set.
- Finish: top with feta and cook 1-2 more minutes. Garnish with herbs. Serve with bread.

Scan to watch

Serves 2

Prep time
10 min

Cook time
30 min

Quick Tips:
- Spicy kick: add extra chili powder or hot sauce for heat.
- Save time: use canned diced tomatoes instead of fresh.
- Impressive serve: serve directly in the skillet
- Green Shakshuka: swap tomatoes for spinach and green bell peppers for a fresh, veggie-packed twist.

Calories: 350 | Protein: 30g | Carbs: 30g | Fats: 20g

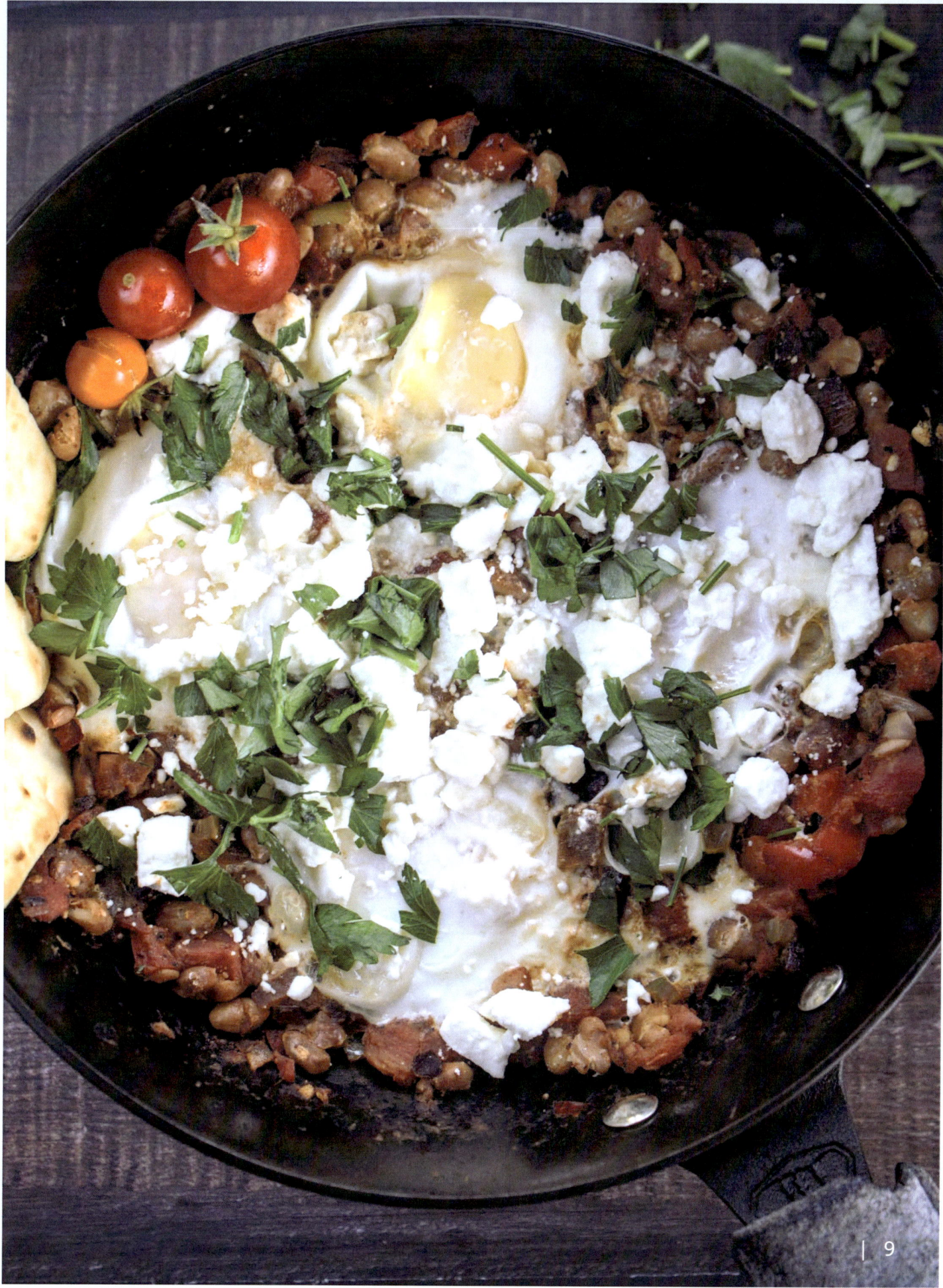

PROTEIN-PACKED AIR FRYER BREAKFAST SANDWICH WITH COTTAGE CHEESE FLATBREAD

Start your day right with this high-protein, filling breakfast sandwich featuring a cottage cheese flatbread. Perfect for a pre-workout meal or to fuel your morning!

Ingredients

For the Flatbread:
- 1/2 cup cottage cheese (14g protein)
- 1 large egg (6g protein)
- 1/4 tsp garlic powder
- 1/4 tsp chili powder
- Salt and pepper, to taste
- 1/4 cup shredded cheddar cheese (5g protein)
- Olive oil spray

For the Sandwich:
- 1 large egg (6g protein)
- 2 slices ham or turkey (10g protein)
- 1/4 avocado, sliced
- Arugula
- 2 tomato slices
- Salt and pepper to taste
- Sriracha to taste

Instructions

- Make the flatbread: in a bowl, mix cottage cheese, egg, garlic powder, seasonings, and cheddar cheese. Spread the mixture on parchment paper in the air fryer sprayed with olive oil. Air fry at 350°F for 15 minutes, until golden and set. Let cool slightly.
- Cook the egg: cook the egg to your preference (scrambled, fried, or poached).
- Assemble the sandwich: place one flatbread on a surface. Spread sriracha, then layer with ham, egg, avocado, arugula, and tomato. Top with the second flatbread.
- Serve: slice and enjoy your high-protein breakfast sandwich!

Scan to watch

Serves 1

Prep time 5 min

Cook time 20 min

Quick Tips:
- For extra flavor: add a sprinkle of smoked paprika or fresh herbs to the flatbread.
- Make it your own: swap ham or turkey for chicken or bacon.
- Meal prep: prepare the flatbread ahead of time and store it in the fridge for a quick sandwich later.

Calories: 470 | Protein: 41g | Carbs: 16g | Fats: 30g

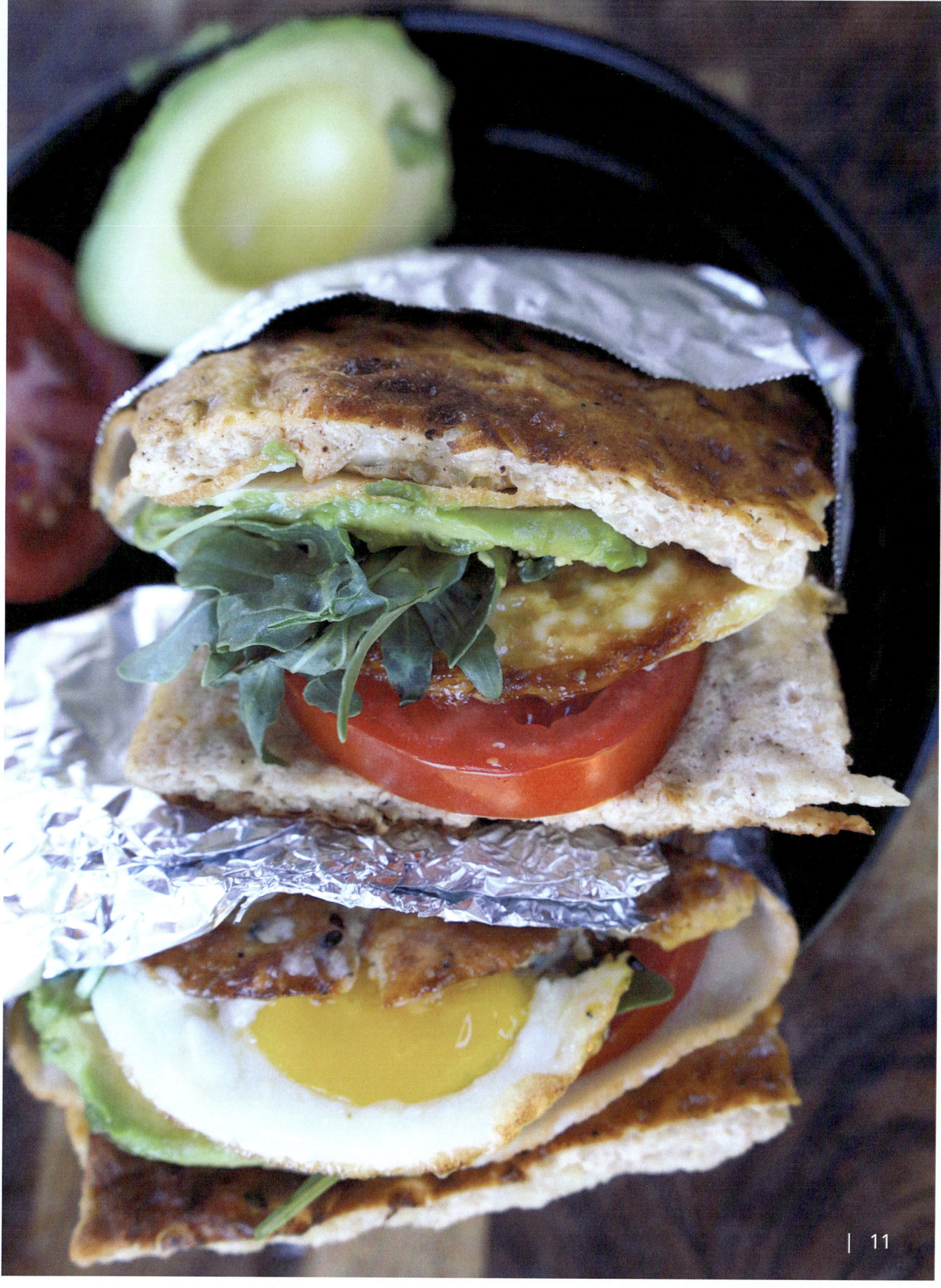

AIR FRYER STUFFED BELL PEPPERS WITH HIGH-PROTEIN BREAKFAST FILLING

Bell peppers are transformed into a hearty, cheesy vessel for a high-protein breakfast filling in this easy air fryer recipe. Perfect for a filling meal that combines cottage cheese, eggs, ham, and garbanzo beans.

Ingredients

Stuffed Bell Peppers:
- 2 large bell peppers
- 2 large eggs
- 1 cup cottage cheese
- 1/2 cup chopped ham
- 1/2 cup garbanzo beans
- Salt and pepper, to taste
- 1/4 tsp ranch seasoning blend
- 1/4 tsp garlic powder
- 1/2 cup chopped green scallions, parsley, dill
- Oil spray

Sauce (Optional):
- Store-bought zhoug sauce or Greek yogurt

Instructions

- Prepare peppers: slice bell peppers horizontally and remove the seeds.
- Make the filling: in a bowl, combine eggs, cottage cheese, ham, garbanzo beans, salt, pepper, ranch seasoning, garlic powder, and chopped herbs.
- Stuff the peppers: spray the bell peppers with oil, then fill with the prepared mixture.
- Cook: air fry at 350°F for 20 minutes, until the peppers are tender and the filling is set.
- Serve: enjoy with zhoug sauce or Greek yogurt.

Scan to watch

Serves 2

Prep time 5 min

Cook time 20 min

Quick Tips:
- Customize the filling: add spinach, mushrooms, or other veggies for extra nutrition.
- For extra flavor: top with shredded cheese or hot sauce before air frying.
- Meal prep: these stuffed peppers can be made ahead and reheated in the air fryer.

Calories: 310 | Protein: 25g | Carbs: 15g | Fats: 18g

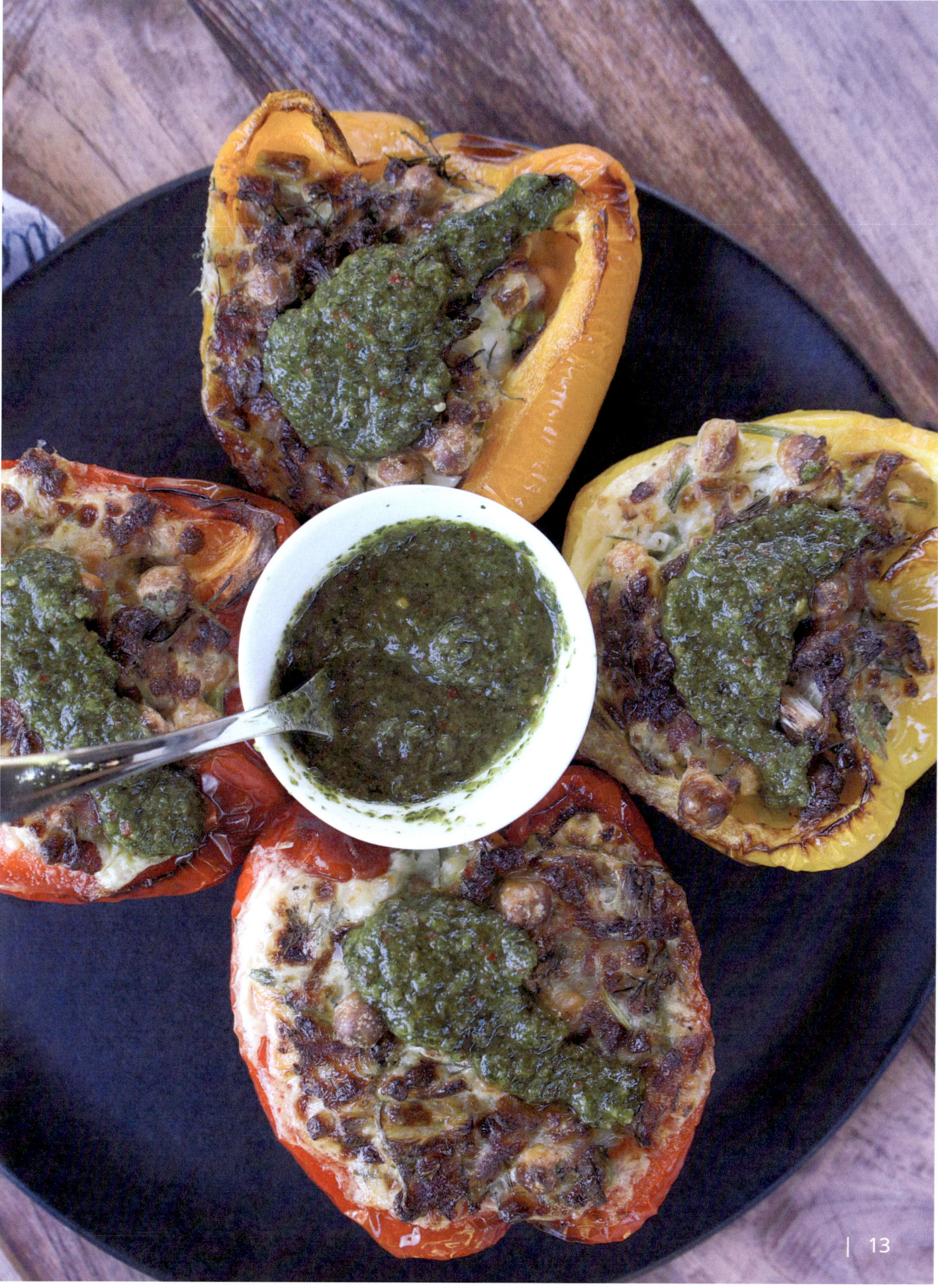

EGG IN A HOLE BREAKFAST SANDWICH

A quick and protein-packed breakfast sandwich inspired by my wife's long-time favorite. The classic "egg in a hole" concept—also known as "egg in a basket"—dates back to the early 20th century. This modern twist adds veggies, cheese, and ham for a complete morning meal.

Ingredients

- **2 slices of bread**
- **1 egg**
- **1/2 bell pepper, chopped**
- **1/2 jalapeño, chopped**
- **1/4 tomato, chopped**
- **1 tbsp green scallions, chopped**
- **1/4 cup Gruyère cheese, shredded**
- **1/2 cup ham, diced**
- **1 tbsp oil**
- **Salt, pepper, seasoning to taste**
- **Ketchup or sriracha for serving**

Instructions

- Prep: cut a square hole in each slice of bread (leave a 1/2-inch border).
- Fry: heat oil in a skillet, stack bread slices, and crack an egg into the hole. Season as desired.
- Fill: add bell pepper, jalapeño, tomatoes, scallions, cheese, and ham into the hole. Top with cut-out bread squares, pressing gently.
- Cook: flip when egg sets, frying the other side for 2-3 minutes until golden.
- Serve: drizzle with sriracha or ketchup and dig in!

Scan to watch

Serves 1

Prep time 5 min

Cook time 5 min

Quick Tips:
- Switch it up: use turkey sausage or swap Gruyere for cheddar.
- Meal prep: pre-chop veggies to save time in the morning.
- Extra flavor: add a drizzle of hot sauce or salsa before serving.

Calories: 400 | Protein: 30g | Carbs: 20g | Fats: 25g

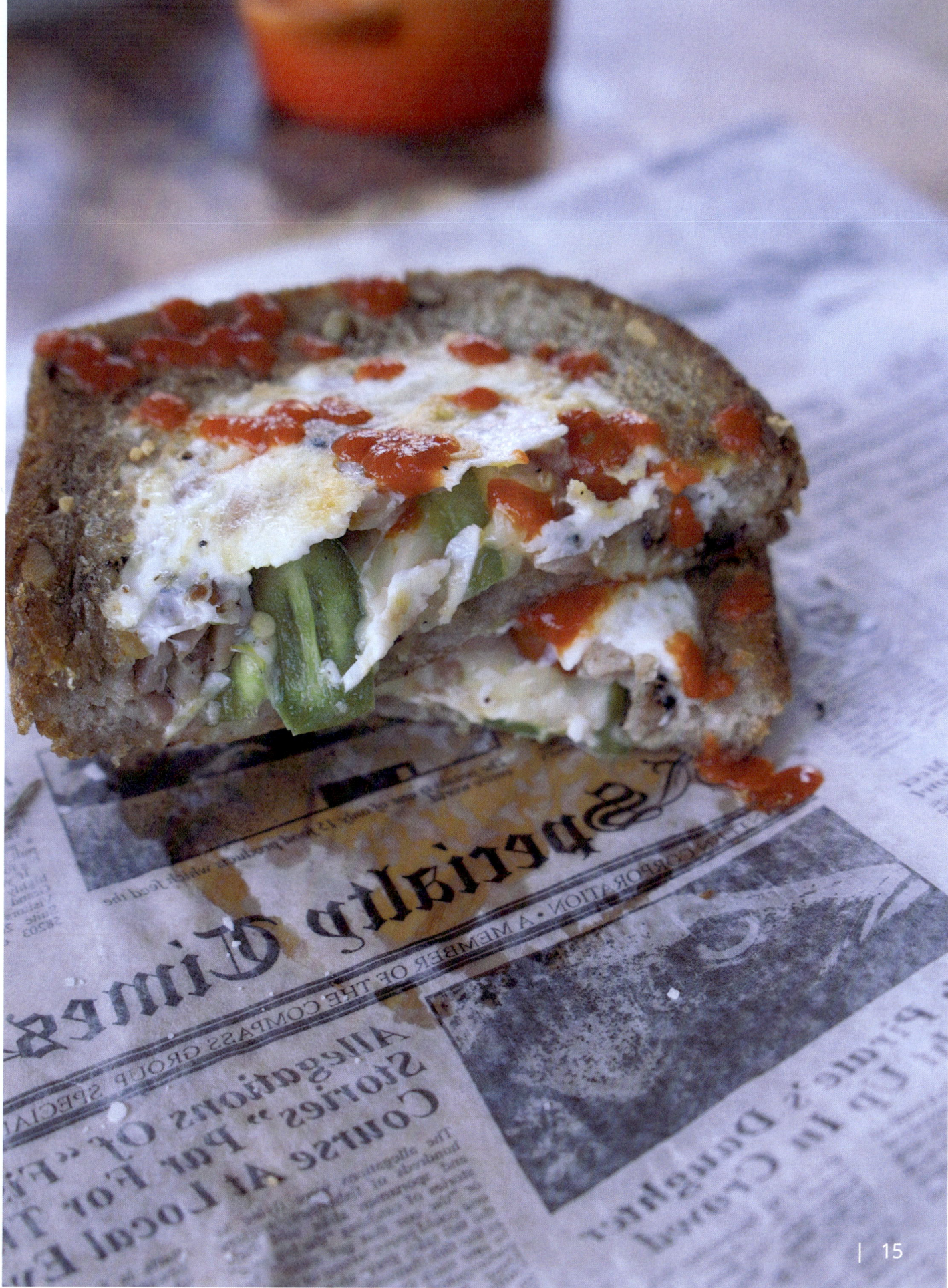

BREAKFAST PIZZA

Pizza for breakfast? Yes, please! This quick, high-protein breakfast pizza is perfect for busy mornings and keeps you fueled for whatever the day throws your way. Customize it with your favorite veggies and proteins!

Ingredients

- **1 low-carb tortilla**
- **2 eggs**
- **1/2 bell pepper, chopped**
- **1/2 jalapeño, chopped**
- **1/4 cup green scallions, chopped**
- **1/2 cup Gruyere cheese, shredded**
- **1/4 cup ham, diced**
- **1/2 cup sausage, chopped**
- **Oil spray**
- **Salt, pepper, chili powder to taste**
- **Optional toppings: pico de gallo and avocado slices**

Instructions

- Preheat: air fryer to 350°F (175°C).
- Assemble: place tortilla in the air fryer basket. Top with bell pepper, jalapeño, scallions, cheese, ham, and sausage.
- Add eggs: crack eggs on top and season.
- Cook: lightly spray with oil. Air fry for 10 minutes or until eggs are set and cheese is melted.
- Serve: slice and top with pico de gallo and avocado if desired.

Scan to watch

Serves 1

Prep time 5 min

Cook time 10 min

Quick Tips:
- Cheese swap: use cheddar or mozzarella if Gruyere isn't available.
- Spice it up: add smoked paprika or chili flakes to the egg.
- Protein boost: swap ham for turkey or add crispy bacon.

Calories: 390 | Protein: 28g | Carbs: 32g | Fats: 16g

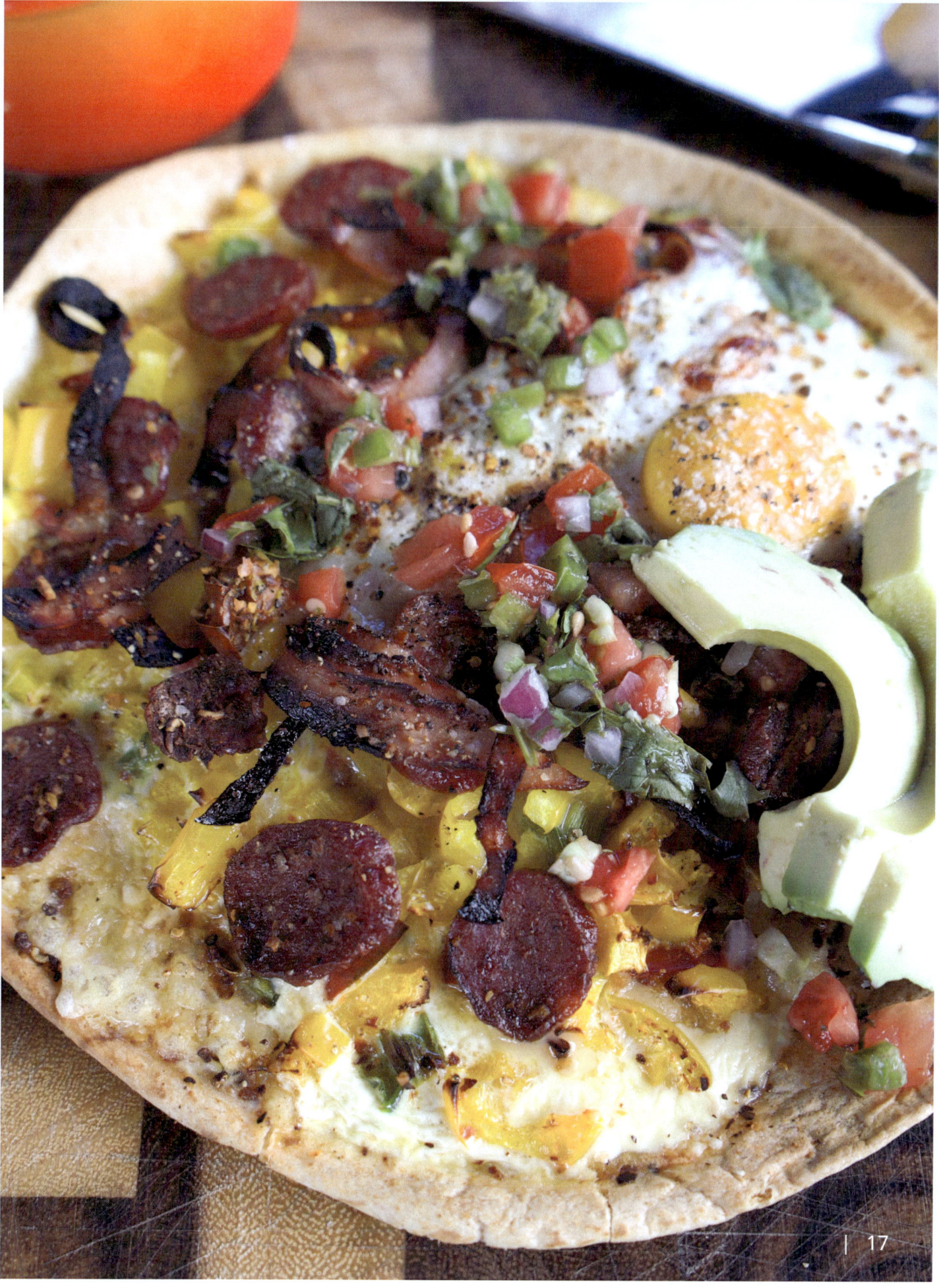

GREEN PROTEIN JUICE WITH COTTAGE CHEESE, YOGURT & PINEAPPLE

My friends are absolutely hooked on this green protein juice. They swear it's the secret to their endless energy and glowing skin. At first, I thought they were just hyping it up—but after trying it myself, I get it. It's creamy, refreshing, and packed with protein.

Ingredients

- **1 cup fresh spinach**
- **1/2 cup pineapple chunks (fresh or frozen)**
- **1/2 green apple, chopped**
- **1 small cucumber, chopped**
- **1/2 cup whole or low-fat milk (or almond milk)**
- **1/2 cup regular cottage cheese**
- **1/2 cup plain Greek yogurt**
- **1 tbsp chia seeds**
- **Juice of 1/2 lemon**
- **Ice cubes (optional)**

Instructions

- Prep ingredients: wash and chop everything.
- Blend: combine all ingredients in a blender and blend until smooth. Adjust thickness with more milk if needed.
- Serve: pour over ice and enjoy the protein-packed goodness.

Scan to watch

Serves 1

Prep time 5 min

Cook time 10 min

Quick Tips:
Need it sweeter? Add half a banana or a drizzle of honey.

Calories: 260 | Protein: 28g | Carbs: 30g | Fats: 8g | Fiber: 5g

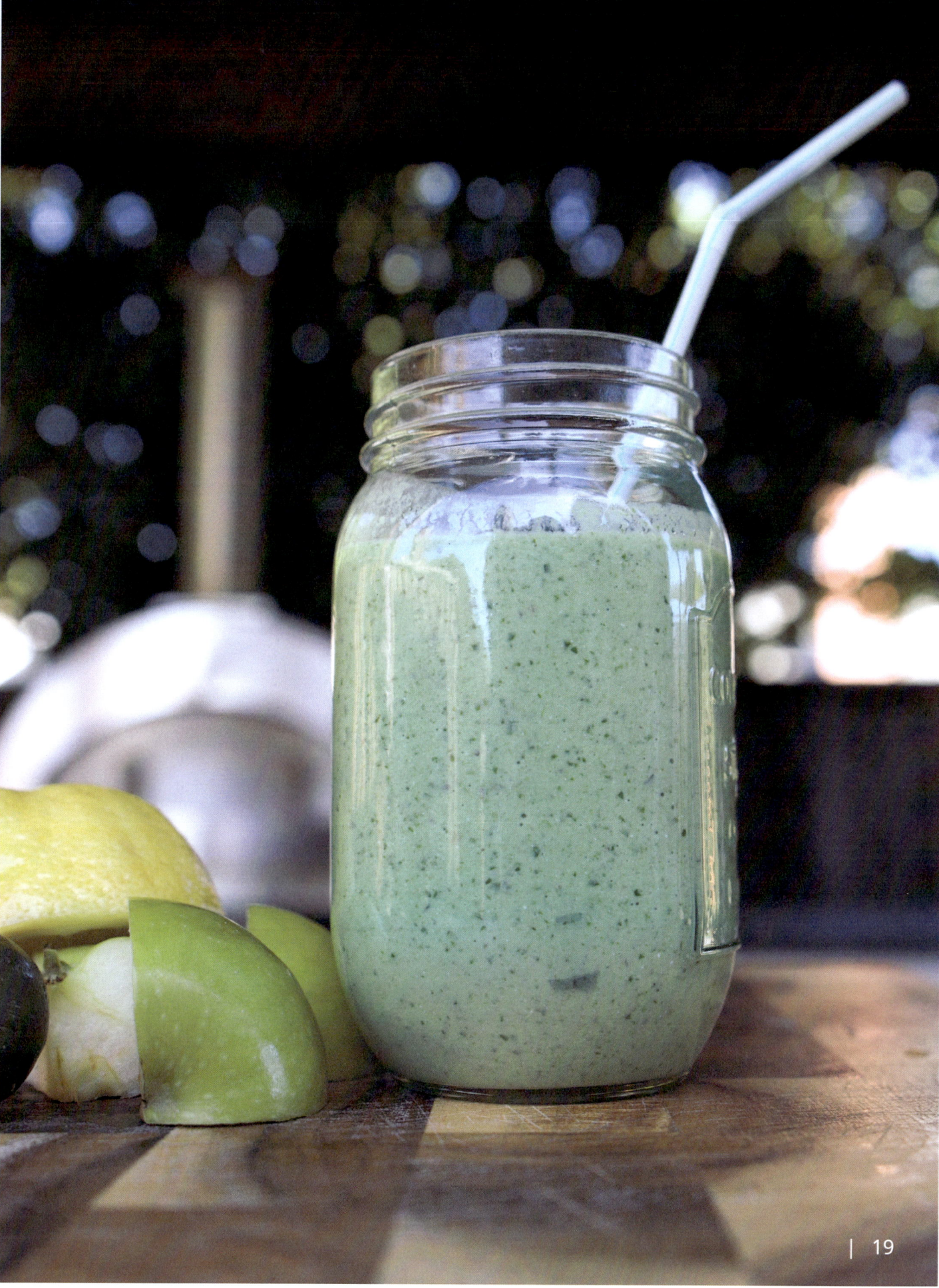

HUEVOS RANCHEROS WITH HIGH-PROTEIN, HEALTHY TWIST

This is my go-to recipe when I want something hearty and flavorful for breakfast or brunch. I love making it on weekends when I have more time to savor a filling meal. I've given the classic huevos rancheros a healthy, high-protein twist while cutting back on fat and carbs, so it aligns perfectly with my healthy eating goals.

Ingredients

- 4 low-carb tortillas
- 1 red onion (chopped)
- 1 jalapeño (chopped)
- 3 cloves garlic (minced)
- 1 can diced tomatoes
- 1/2 cup parsley (chopped)
- Salt & pepper to taste
- 1 tsp cumin powder
- 1 tsp chili powder
- 1/2 lb ground beef
- 4 eggs
- Oil (for sautéing vegetables and meat)
- Oil spray (for air-frying tortillas)
- 1/2 can low-fat refried beans
- Toppings: sriracha sauce, avocado slices, parsley or cilantro, cotija cheese, and crema

Instructions

- Sauté vegetables & beef: in a skillet, heat oil over medium heat. Sauté onions and jalapeño for 3 minutes. Add garlic and cook for 1 minute. Stir in tomatoes, ground beef, cumin, chili powder, salt, and pepper. Cook until beef is browned. Stir in parsley and remove from heat.
- Air-fry tortillas: lightly spray tortillas with oil and air-fry at 350°F for 5 minutes until crispy.
- Cook eggs: prepare eggs to your preferred doneness (fried or scrambled).
- Assemble Rancheros: spread refried beans on each tortilla. Top with ground beef mixture, a cooked egg, and your favorite toppings: sriracha, cotija cheese, avocado, and parsley or cilantro.

Scan to watch

Serves 4

Prep time 15 min

Cook time 20 min

Quick Tips:
- Vegetarian option: use black beans or plant-based protein instead of beef.
- Spice it up: add more jalapeño or hot sauce for extra heat.
- Boost fiber: top with spinach or arugula for added fiber.

Calories: 380 | Protein: 30g | Carbs: 18g | Fats: 24g

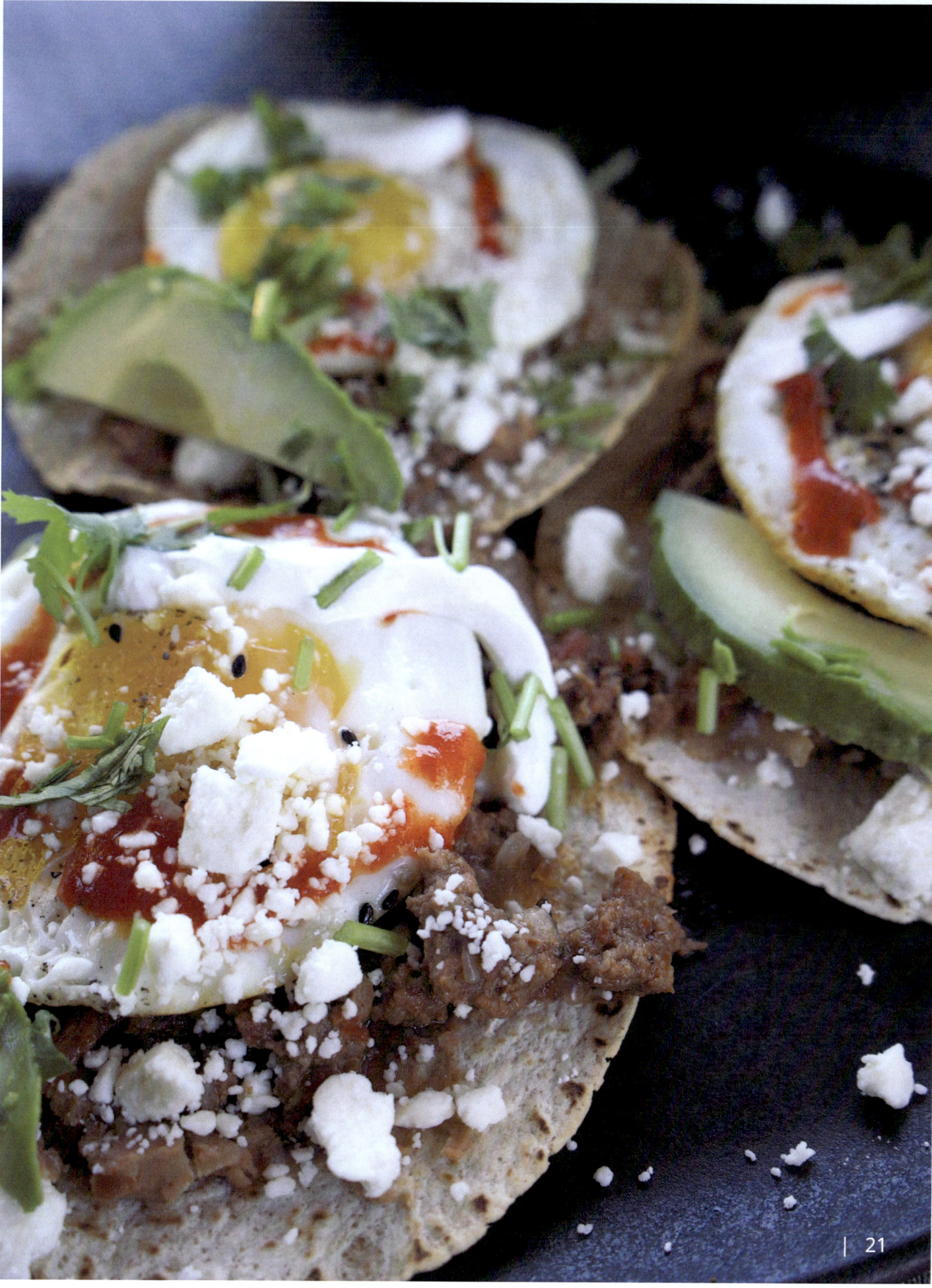

HIGH-PROTEIN EGG BITES

The ultimate meal prep for your mornings! These high-protein egg bites are quick to make, super portable, and packed with all the good stuff to kick-start your day. Oh, and they were a huge hit at the potluck at my gym—everyone loved them! Now, they're a regular in my morning routine. This recipe makes 24 egg bites.

Ingredients

- **12 large eggs**
- **1 bell pepper (chopped)**
- **1 cup mushrooms (chopped)**
- **1 cup sausage & ham (chopped)**
- **2 cups spinach**
- **1½ cups cottage cheese**
- **1 cup chickpeas**
- **1 cup shredded Gruyere cheese**
- **2 tbsp sriracha sauce**
- **Salt & pepper to taste**
- **Oil (for sautéing)**
- **Oil spray (for muffin tin)**

Instructions

- Sauté the ingredients: bell pepper, mushrooms, sausage, ham, and spinach until soft. Set aside.
- Blend the mixture: In a blender, combine eggs, cottage cheese, chickpeas, Gruyere cheese, salt, pepper, and sriracha. Blend until smooth.
- Assemble the egg bites: preheat oven to 325°F. Spray a muffin tin with oil spray. Spoon the sautéed mixture into each cup, then pour egg mixture.
- Bake: place a baking dish of water on the bottom rack to keep egg bites moist. Bake for 25 minutes, or until set.
- Cool and store: let cool slightly before removing from the tin. Store in an airtight container in the fridge for up to a week.

Scan to watch

Serves 12

Prep time 10 min

Cook time 30 min

Quick Tips:
Vegetarian option: use fresh tomatoes and spinach instead of sausage and ham for a veggie-packed version!

Calories: 120 | Protein: 7g | Carbs: 4g | Fats: 8g

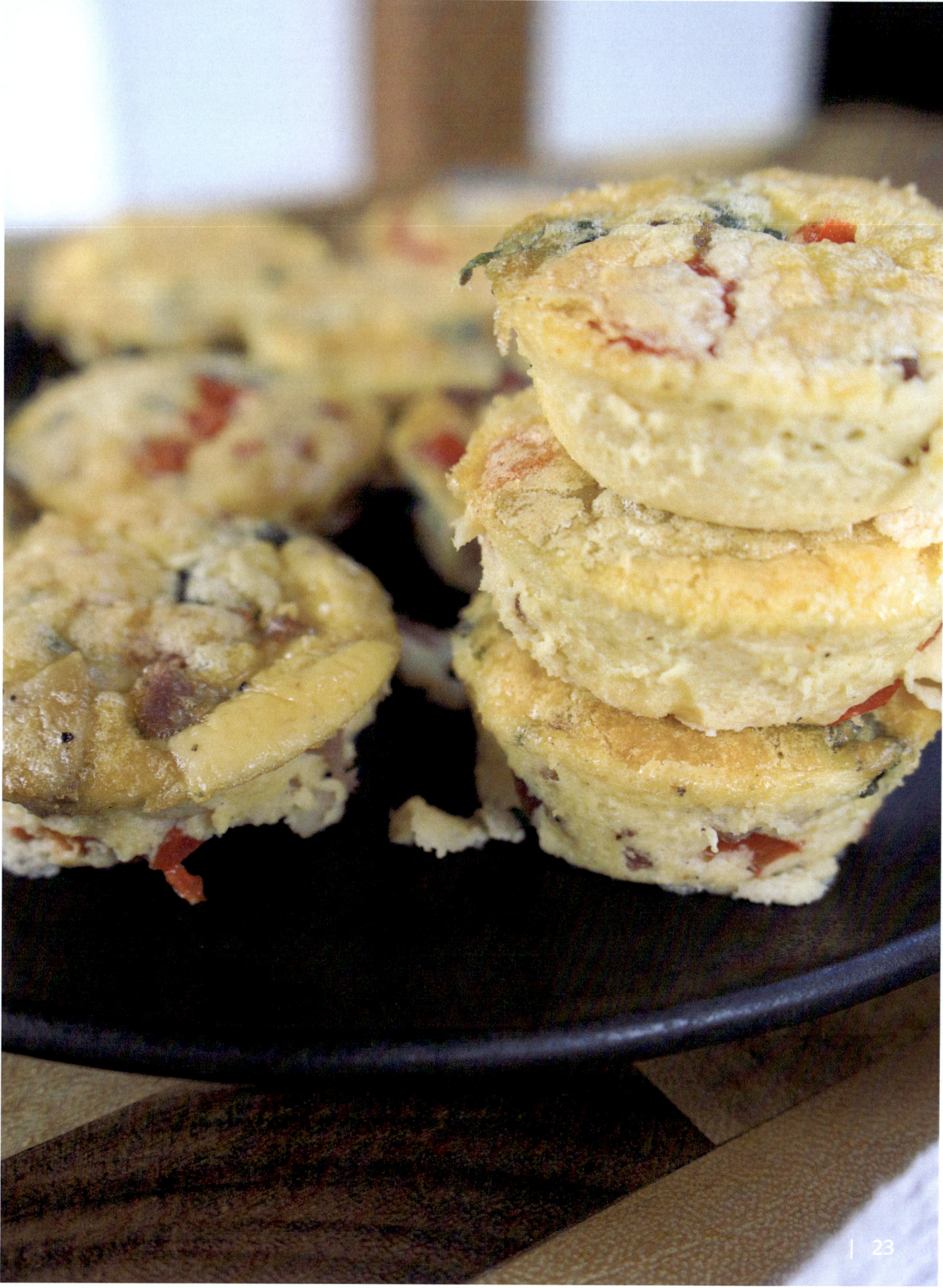

ZUCCHINI BREAKFAST PANCAKES (AND BREAKFAST SANDWICH)

Growing up, zucchini was always a staple in our kitchen, and there are countless ways to turn it into something delicious. These pancakes are the ultimate morning power move, especially if you're gearing up for a workout. Makes 12 pancakes.

Ingredients

- **4 medium zucchinis, shredded (about 1.2 lb after removing water)**
- **1/2 cup cottage cheese**
- **1/2 cup almond or coconut flour**
- **2 large eggs**
- **1/4 cup grated Parmesan cheese**
- **1/2 cup fresh basil, chopped**
- **1 tsp garlic powder**
- **Salt and pepper to taste**
- **Oil for cooking**

Instructions

- Prepare the zucchini: shred zucchinis and squeeze out water using cheesecloth. Add a little salt before draining to help extract more water.
- Mix the ingredients: in a large bowl, combine zucchini, cottage cheese, Parmesan, flour, eggs, basil, garlic powder, salt, and pepper. Mix until thick.
- Cook the pancakes: heat a non-stick skillet over medium heat, lightly coat with oil, and scoop 1 tbsp of batter per pancake. Flatten slightly and cook 3-4 minutes per side until golden. Air Fryer Option: Spray with oil and cook at 350°F for 10-12 minutes, flipping halfway.
- Assemble the sandwich: layer one pancake with Dijon mustard, arugula, tomato, ham, cheese and a cooked egg.

Scan to watch

Serves 4

Prep time 10 min

Cook time 15 min

Quick Tips:
- Add protein powder to the batter for even more protein.
- Make sure zucchini is super dry to avoid soggy pancakes.
- Switch up fillings with turkey bacon or roasted veggies.
- Serve hot or wrap in foil for a grab-and-go breakfast.

Per Pancake: Calories: ~80 | Protein: ~7g | Carbs: ~3g | Fat: ~5g

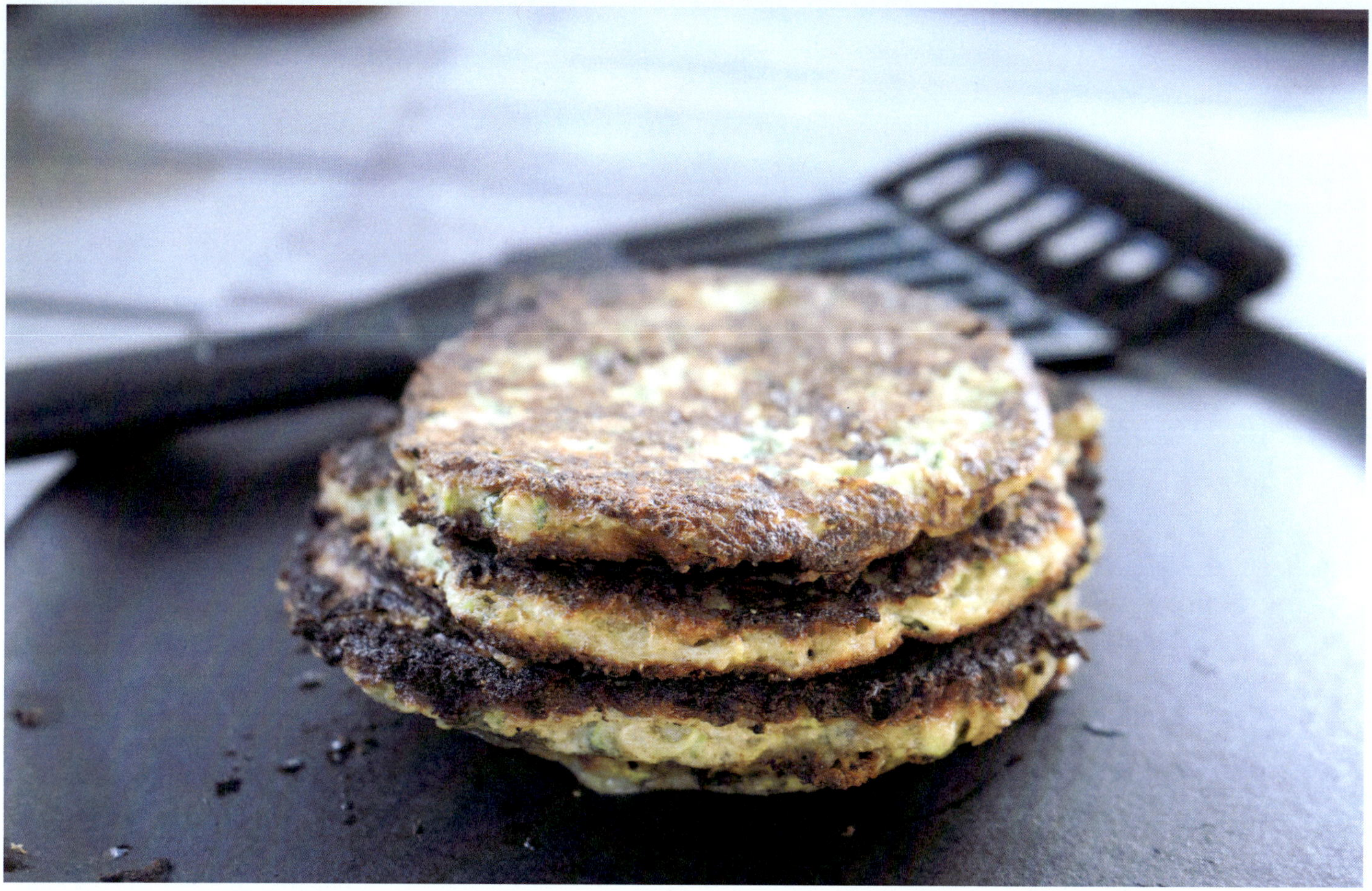

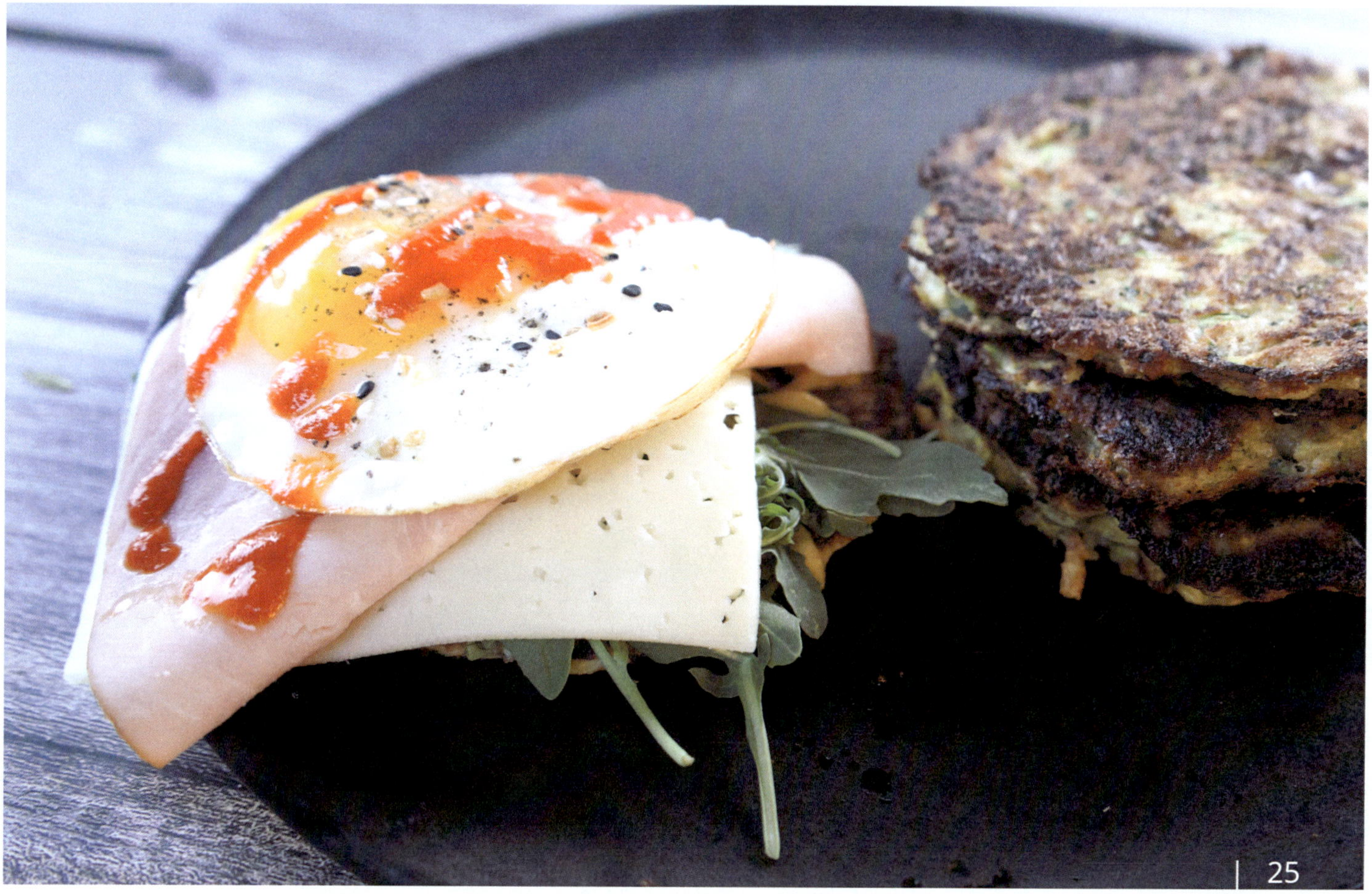

HIGH-PROTEIN LAVASH BREAKFAST WRAPS

Mornings can be chaotic, but these wraps are my secret weapon. Packed with protein, they're easy to make, perfect for meal prep, and keep me full till lunch. Plus, they taste way better than anything store-bought!

Ingredients

Egg mixture:
- 2 (16 oz) packages egg whites
- 2 cups spinach, chopped
- 1 bell pepper, chopped
- 1 smoked sausage, sliced
- ⅔ cup sun-dried tomatoes, chopped
- 1 cup feta cheese
- 1 tsp garlic powder
- 1 tsp onion powder
- Salt & pepper to taste

Wrap assembly:
- 4 lavash bread sheets
- ½ cup cream cheese
- Oil for toasting
- Oil spray

Instructions

- Preheat oven to 375°F. Spray a baking dish with oil and line with parchment paper.
- Pour egg whites into the dish. Top evenly with spinach, bell pepper, sausage, sun-dried tomatoes, seasonings, and feta.
- Bake for 25 minutes or until set. Let cool slightly and cut into 4 portions.
- Spread cream cheese on each lavash. Add one egg portion per wrap.
- Fold and toast in a skillet with oil until crispy on both sides.
- Slice in half and serve hot.

Scan to watch

Serves 8

Prep time
10 min

Cook time
25 min

Quick Tips:
- Freezer-friendly: wrap and freeze. Reheat in the microwave and finish in a skillet.
- Swap ingredients: use turkey bacon, tofu, or different cheese for variety.

Per Wrap: Calories: ~275 | Protein: ~23g | Carbs: ~20g | Fat: ~12g

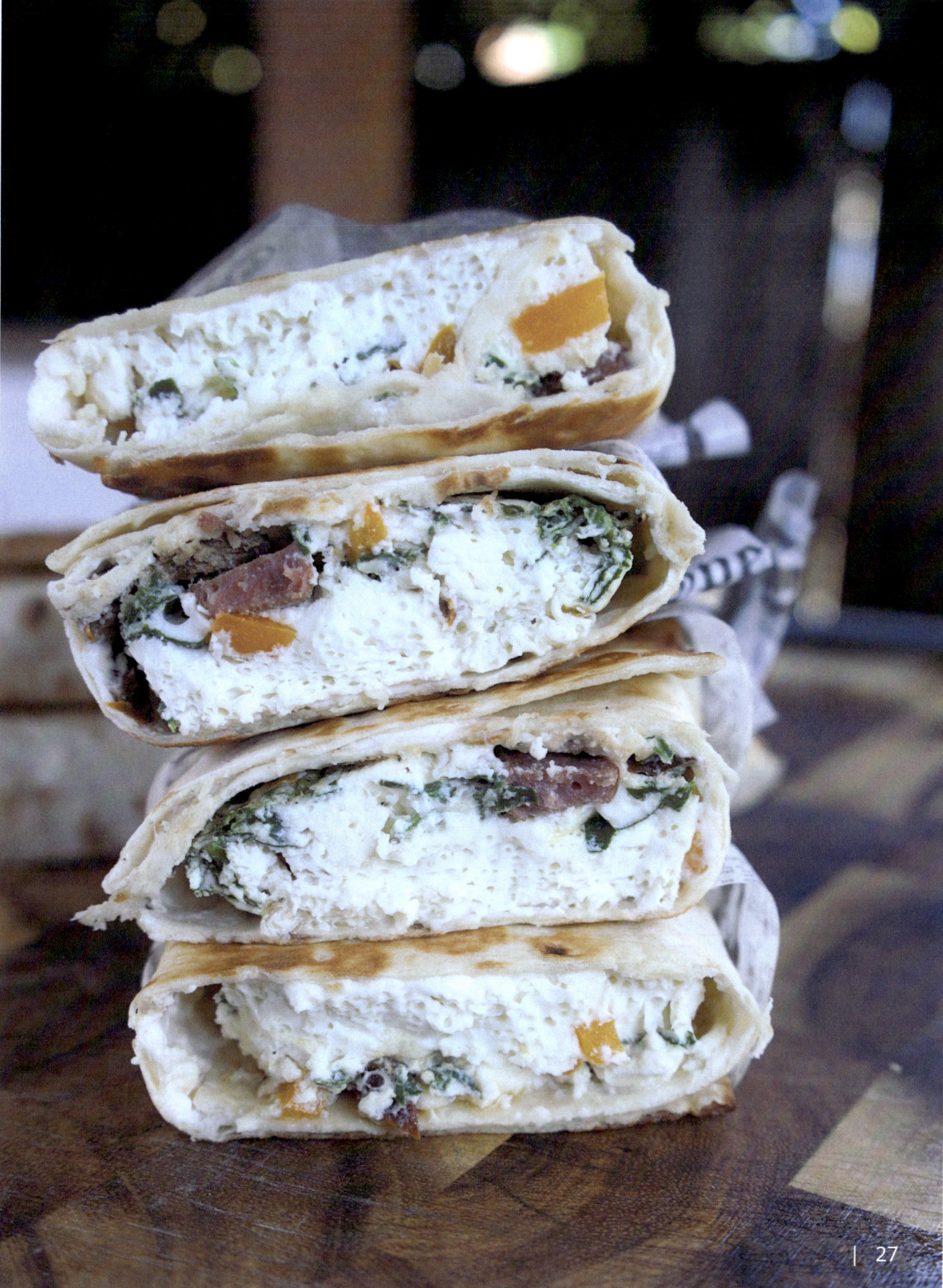

BULK-BATCH BREAKFAST BURRITOS

These breakfast burritos are made for real life—easy to prep, freezer-friendly, and packed with enough protein to actually keep you full. I make a batch at the start of the week, and mornings instantly run smoother. They're also versatile enough to tweak depending on what's in your fridge

Ingredients

- **7 potatoes — boiled (Instant Pot: 10 min manual)**
- **2 bell peppers — sliced**
- **1 cup cherry tomatoes — sliced**
- **3 cups arugula**
- **1 lb ground beef — seasoned with 1 tsp salt, ½ tsp pepper, pinch of cumin**
- **2 cups shredded Mexican cheese blend**
- **6 eggs — beaten and seasoned**
- **Olive oil — for the skillet**
- **10 low-carb tortillas**

Instructions

- Boil the potatoes: Instant Pot for 10 minutes (manual). Let cool, then cube.
- Prep the baking dish: lightly oil a 10x14" dish. Layer half the cubed potatoes, then top with bell peppers and cherry tomatoes. Season lightly.
- Add greens and beef: spread arugula over veggies, add cooked ground beef, and top with the rest of the veggies. Season again.
- Add cheese and eggs: sprinkle shredded cheese evenly. Pour beaten eggs over the top.
- Bake: 380°F for 30–35 minutes until set.
- Wrap the burritos: slice baked mixture into 10 portions. Stuff each into a tortilla and roll tightly.
- Grill: crisp up each burrito in an oiled skillet until golden on both sides.

Scan to watch

10 Burritos

Prep time
20 min

Cook time
35 min

Quick Tips:
- Great with avocado, hot sauce, or extra salsa.
- Swap ground beef for turkey, chicken, or plant-based crumbles. Add black beans for extra fiber.
- Wrap each burrito individually in foil and freeze.

Calories: 320 | Protein: 25g | Carbs: 20g | Fat: 16g

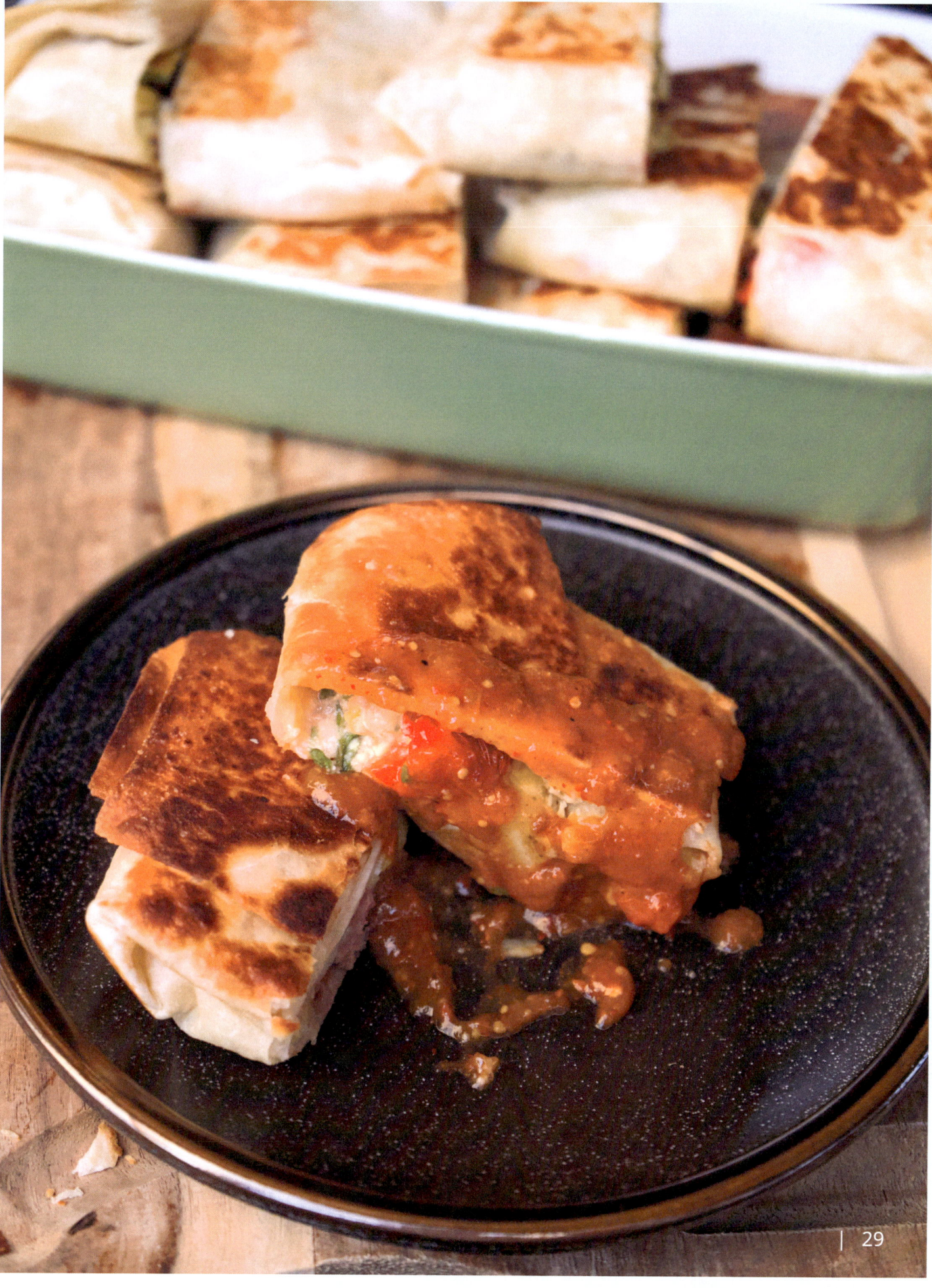

You've had your eggs and protein waffles.
Now it's time for a little comfort-in-a-bowl therapy.

Let the soups and stews begin.

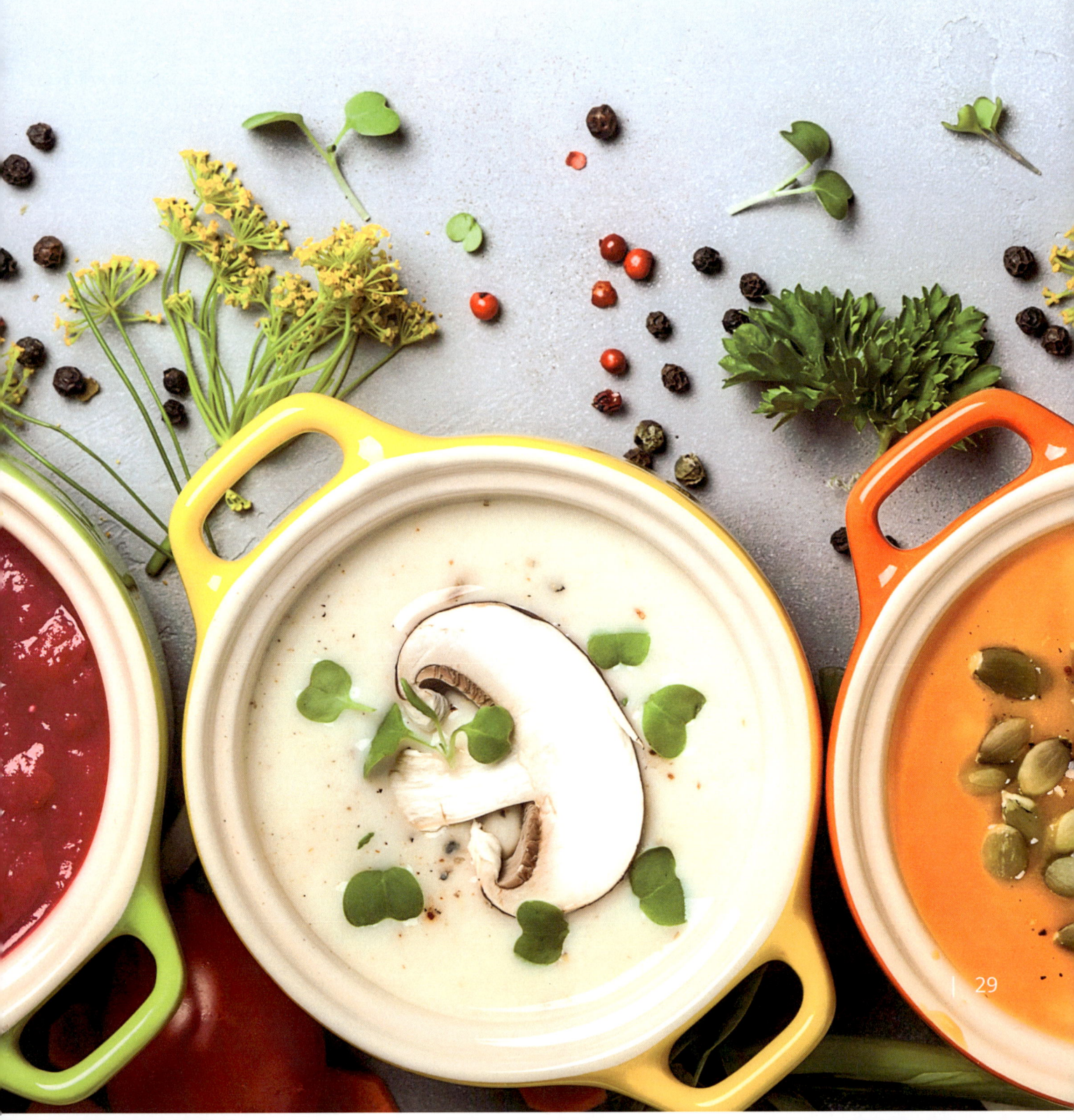

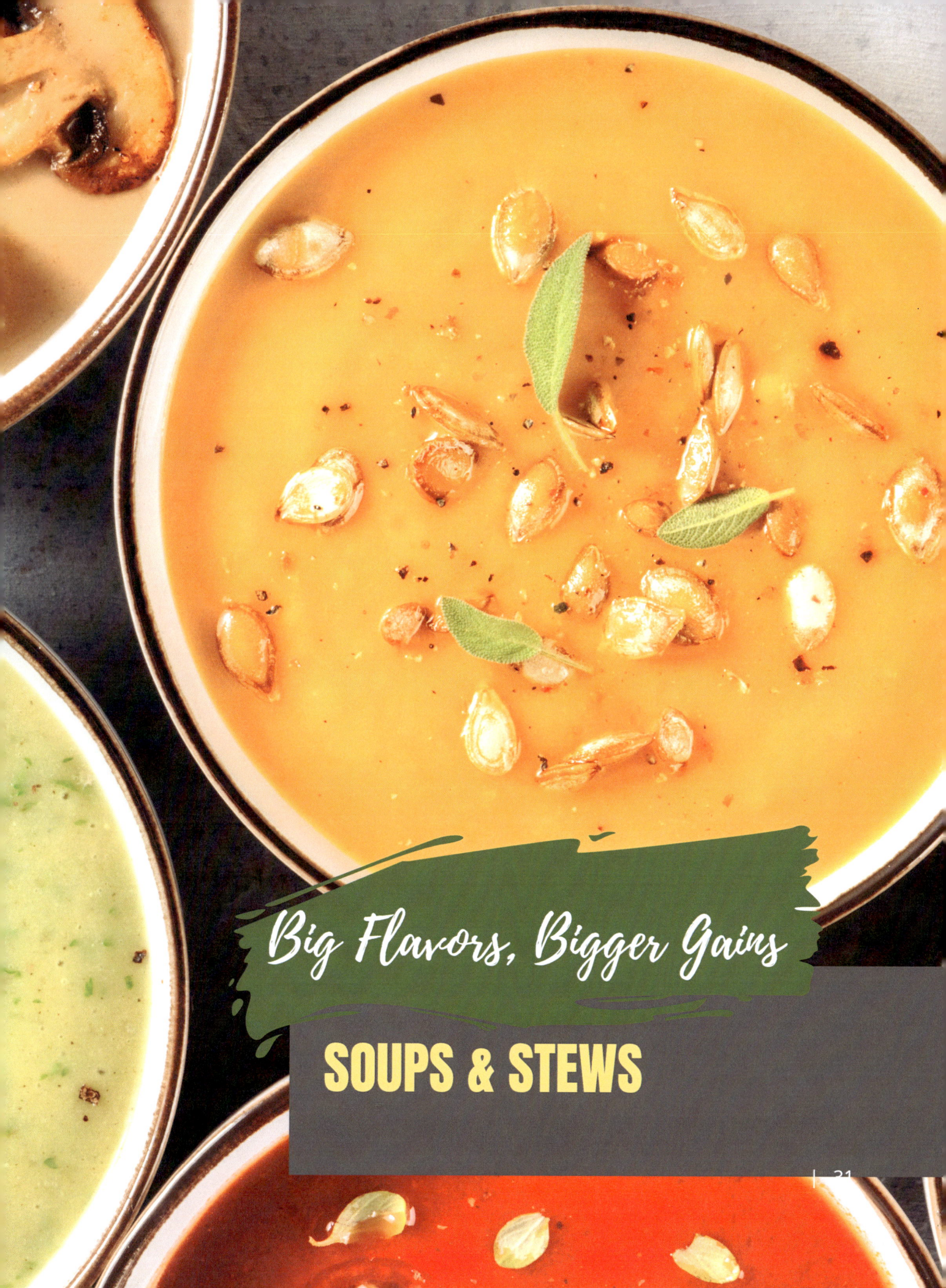

Big Flavors, Bigger Gains

SOUPS & STEWS

CAN'T RESIST CHICKPEAS

This dish is one of my all-time favorite high-protein meals. It's easy to make, filling, and packed with vitamins and nutrients. Plus, it's made entirely with pantry ingredients—perfect for a quick, satisfying lunch or dinner!

Ingredients

- **1 onion, chopped**
- **3 garlic cloves, minced**
- **2 tomatoes, diced**
- **2 tbsp tomato paste**
- **½ cup sun-dried tomatoes**
- **2 cans (15 oz each) chickpeas, drained**
- **1 can (14 oz) coconut milk**
- **Juice of ½ lime**
- **2 tbsp fruit vinegar (like blueberry vinegar)**
- **8 cups kale**
- **Oregano, salt, and pepper to taste**
- **Oil for sautéing**

Instructions

- Sauté onion & garlic: heat oil in a skillet over medium heat. Sauté onion for 5 minutes until soft, then add garlic and sauté 2 more minutes.
- Add tomatoes & flavor: stir in diced tomatoes, tomato paste, and sun-dried tomatoes. Cook for 5 minutes until tomatoes soften.
- Combine & simmer: add chickpeas, coconut milk, lime juice, vinegar, oregano, salt, and pepper. Simmer on medium-low for 15 minutes.
- Finish with kale: add kale and cook for 5 more minutes, until wilted and tender.
- Serve: dish up with your favorite bread, pita, or naan.

Scan to watch

Serves 4

Prep time 10 min

Cook time 20 min

Quick Tips:
- No kale? Swap with spinach or Swiss chard.
- Make it spicier with red pepper flakes or smoked paprika.
- Use canned diced tomatoes.

Calories: ~365 | Protein: ~15g | Carbs: ~38g | Fat: ~18g | Fiber: ~11g

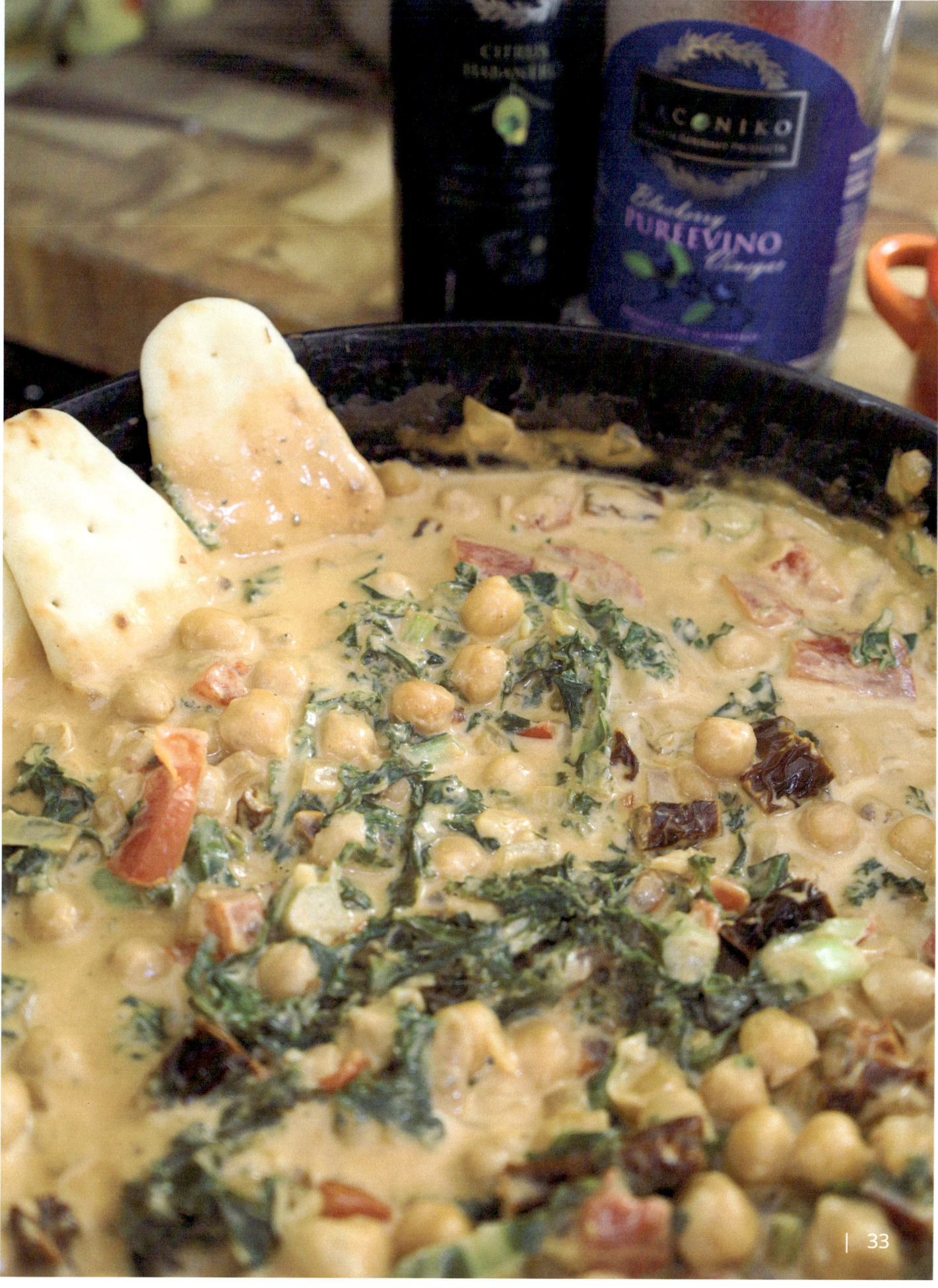

INSTANT POT CHILI

This Instant Pot chili is the ultimate comfort food, packed with savory, spicy, and sweet flavors. Top it with a golden cornbread layer, and you've got a dish that's both hearty and satisfying. Plus, it's perfect for ski trips—just pop it in the Instant Pot, and it'll stay warm all day, ready to enjoy after a long day on the slopes.

Ingredients

- **1 lb ground beef (or any other ground meat)**
- **1 ½ cups diced bacon**
- **1 red onion, chopped**
- **1 jalapeño, chopped**
- **3 cloves garlic, minced**
- **3 cans beans (northern beans, pinto beans, kidney beans)**
- **2 ½ tbsp molasses**
- **1 tbsp brown sugar**
- **2 ½ tbsp tomato paste**
- **1 tbsp worcestershire sauce**
- **1 tbsp apple cider vinegar**
- **Juice of 1 lime**
- **¼ cup dark chocolate**
- **1 red chili pepper, chopped**
- **Salt & pepper to taste**

Instructions

- Prep the bacon & veggies: set your Instant Pot to sauté mode. Add diced bacon and cook until crispy. Remove the bacon but leave the fat in the pot. Add the ground beef to the bacon fat and cook until browned halfway. Stir in red onion, cooking for 3 minutes, followed by the jalapeño, garlic, salt, pepper, and apple cider vinegar.
- Build the chili base: add the beans, cooked bacon, molasses, brown sugar, tomato paste, worcestershire sauce, lime juice, red chili pepper, and dark chocolate to the pot. Mix everything together.
- Pressure cook: select manual or pressure cook on high for 15 minutes. Allow a natural pressure release.

Scan to watch

Serves 6

Prep time
15 min

Cook time
30 min

Quick Tips:
- Top your chili with cornbread! Prepare cornbread from a package and bake it on top of the chili.
- Take this chili to the ski resort inside your Instant Pot—it stays warm all day, making it the perfect meal after a day on the slopes!

Without cornbread topping: Calories: 650 | Protein: 35g | Carbs: 50g | Fat: 35g

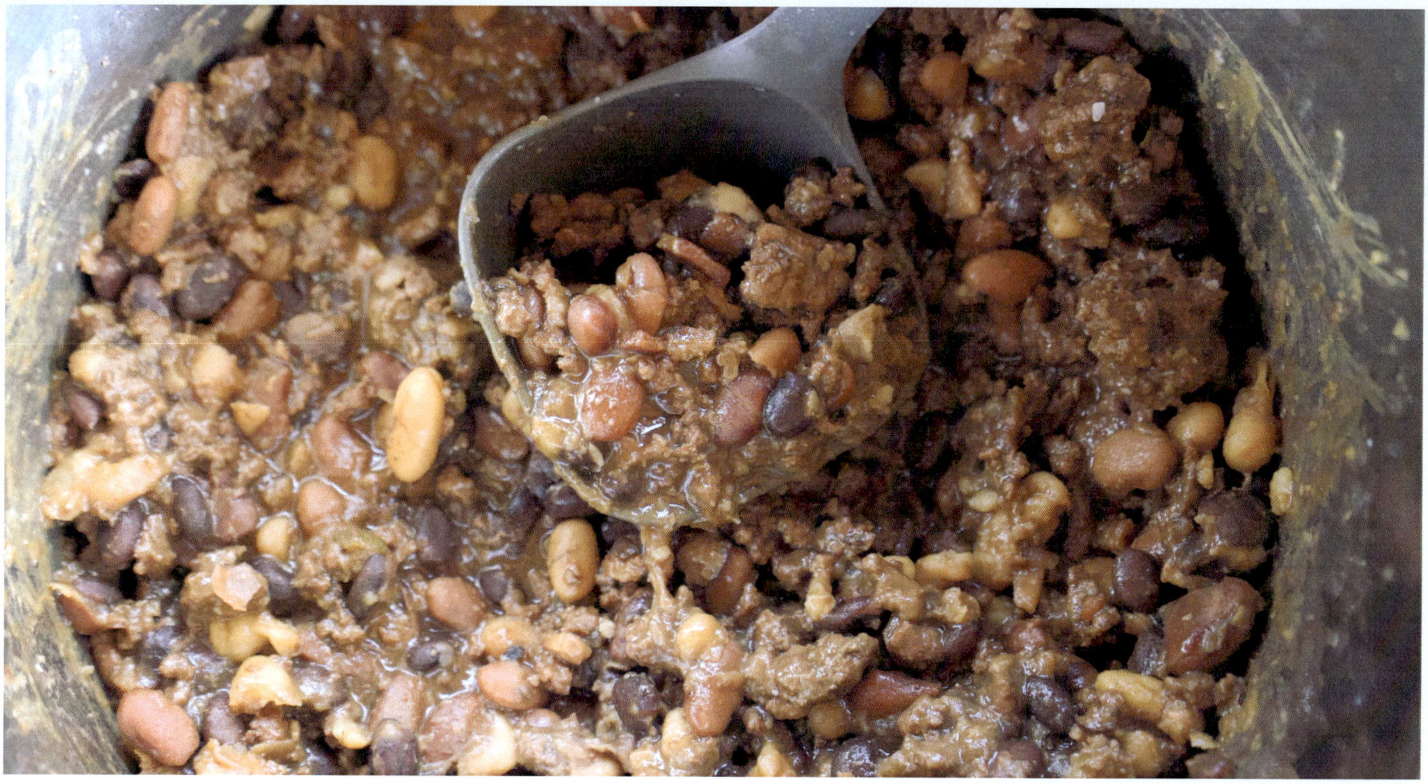

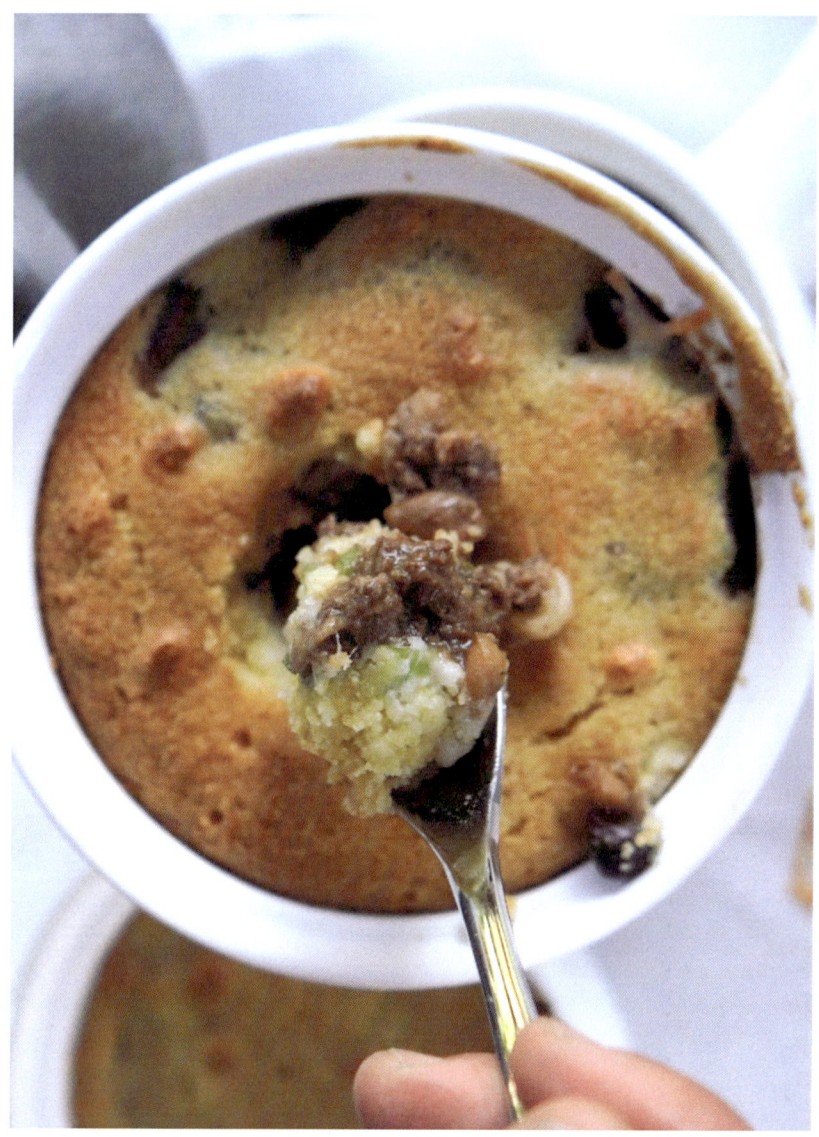
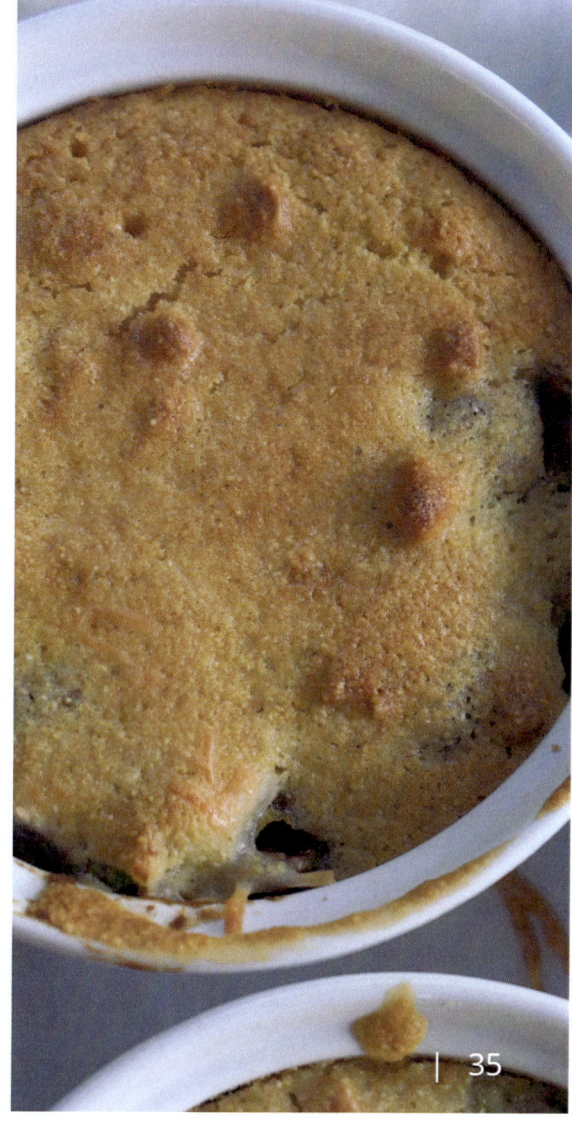

TACO SOUP – INSTANT POT STYLE

Craving something warm, hearty, and protein-packed? This Taco Soup with a Fall Twist delivers all the spicy goodness of tacos with a cozy butternut squash upgrade—ready in under 30 minutes. Meal-prep friendly, satisfying, and perfect for chilly days!

Ingredients

- **1 lb (450g) lean ground turkey or beef**
- **2 cups butternut squash, cubed (divided)**
- **1 zucchini, diced**
- **1 small onion, diced**
- **2 bell peppers, chopped**
- **1 jalapeño, chopped**
- **3 garlic cloves, minced**
- **1 can (14 oz) diced tomatoes**
- **1 can (15 oz) black beans, drained & rinsed**
- **½ cup corn**
- **1 ½ cups chicken or beef broth (low sodium)**
- **1 tbsp olive oil**
- **½ packet taco seasoning**
- **1 tsp cumin**
- **1 tsp smoked paprika**
- **Salt & pepper to taste**

Optional toppings: shredded cheese, avocado, cilantro, Greek yogurt, roasted squash, jalapeños, balsamic glaze

Instructions

- Sauté: set Instant Pot to sauté mode. Heat olive oil, cook onions and jalapeño for 5 min, then add garlic.
- Brown the meat: add ground turkey (or beef) and cook until browned.
- Add veggies & beans: stir in tomatoes, black beans, corn, zucchini, and half the butternut squash.
- Season & simmer: add taco seasoning, cumin, smoked paprika, salt, and pepper. Pour in broth, seal the lid, and cook on high pressure for 12 minutes.
- Release & serve: quick-release pressure, stir, and adjust seasoning. Serve with toppings and the reserved roasted butternut squash.

Scan to watch

Serves 4

Prep time 10 min

Cook time 20 min

Quick Tips:
- Use the Instant Pot lid while sautéing to trap heat and soften onions faster.
- Deglaze the pot with a splash of broth after browning meat to avoid stuck bits triggering a burn warning.

Calories: 280 | Protein: 28g | Carbs: 22g | Fat: 10g

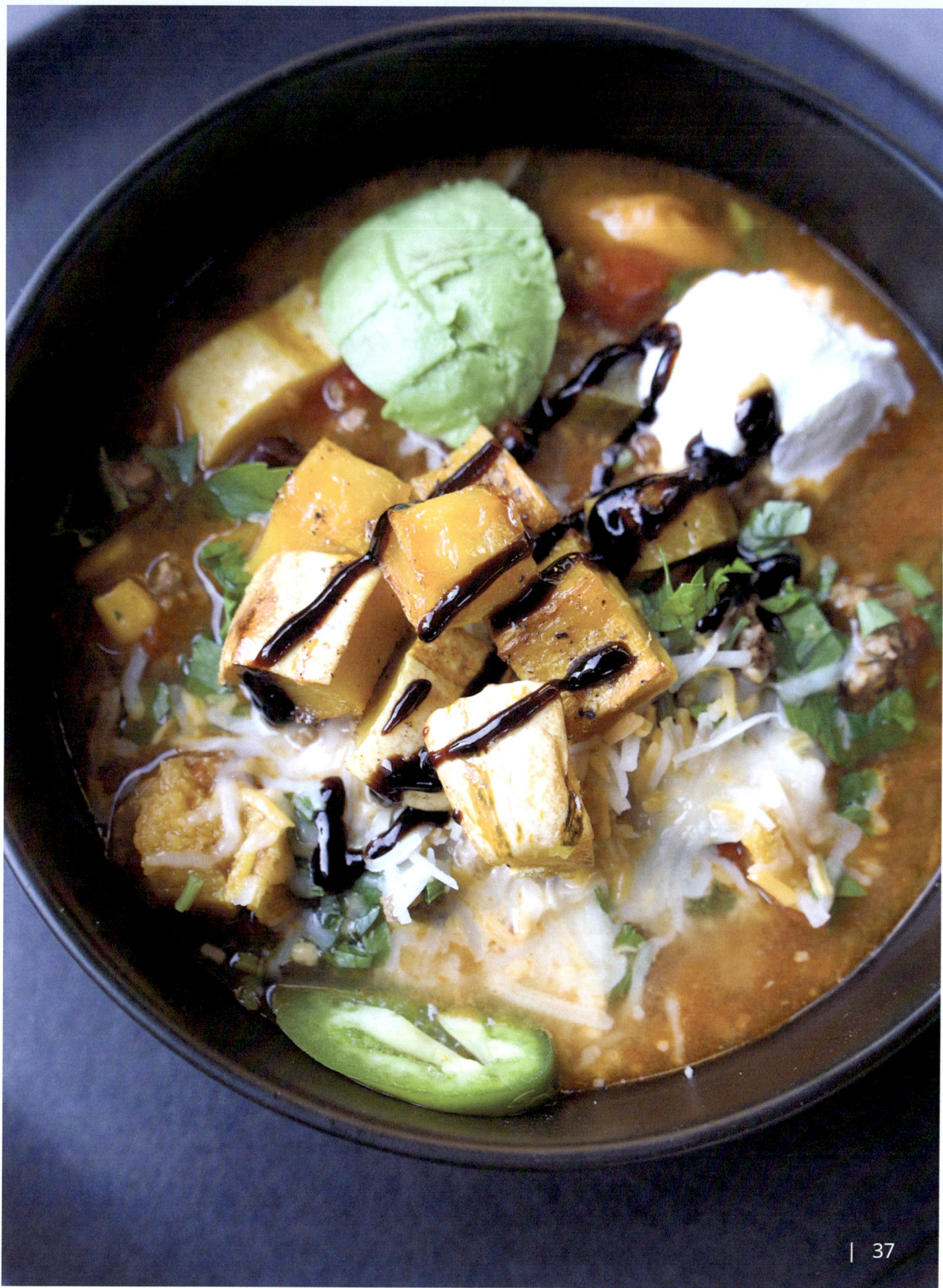

CAULIFLOWER, CASHEWS AND CHICKPEAS SOUP

A rich and creamy fall soup made with cashews and chickpeas, creating a velvety texture without any cream or extra fat. Made easy with the Instant Pot for a one-pot, hassle-free meal.

Ingredients

- **1 onion, chopped**
- **3 garlic cloves, minced**
- **1 cup mushrooms, chopped**
- **1 head cauliflower, florets**
- **1 can chickpeas, divided**
- **1 cup cashews, soaked**
- **2 cups potatoes, cubed**
- **1 cup coconut milk**
- **1 tbsp chicken broth**
- **Zest & juice of 1 lemon**
- **1 tsp cheesy seasoning blend**
- **1 tsp paprika**
- **1 tsp cinnamon**
- **1 tsp chili powder**
- **Salt & pepper to taste**
- **1 tbsp Oil (for sautéing)**

Toppings:
- **Extra virgin olive oil**
- **Balsamic glaze**
- **Fresh dill**
- **Roasted chickpeas**

Instructions

- Sauté: set Instant Pot to Sauté. Heat oil and sauté onion for 3 minutes. Add garlic, cook 1 more minute.
- Cook: add mushrooms, cauliflower, ½ can chickpeas, soaked cashews, potatoes, coconut milk, chicken broth, lemon zest, lemon juice, and spices. Stir well.
- Pressure cook: seal lid, cook on manual pressure for 10 minutes. After 5-minute natural release.
- Blend: use a handheld blender to purée until smooth. Adjust seasoning as needed.
- Roast chickpeas: toss remaining chickpeas in oil and seasoning. Roast at 400°F for 15-20 minutes.
- Serve: ladle soup into bowls. Top with olive oil, balsamic glaze, fresh dill, and roasted chickpeas.

Scan to watch

Serves 4

Prep time 10 min

Cook time 25 min

Quick Tips:
- Soak cashews ahead of time or use boiling water for a quick soak (10-15 minutes) to soften.
- If soup is too thin, blend in more of the cauliflower and potatoes.
- This soup freezes well. Store in airtight containers for up to 3 months!

Calories: 529 | Protein: 17.6g | Carbs: 50g | Fat: 28g

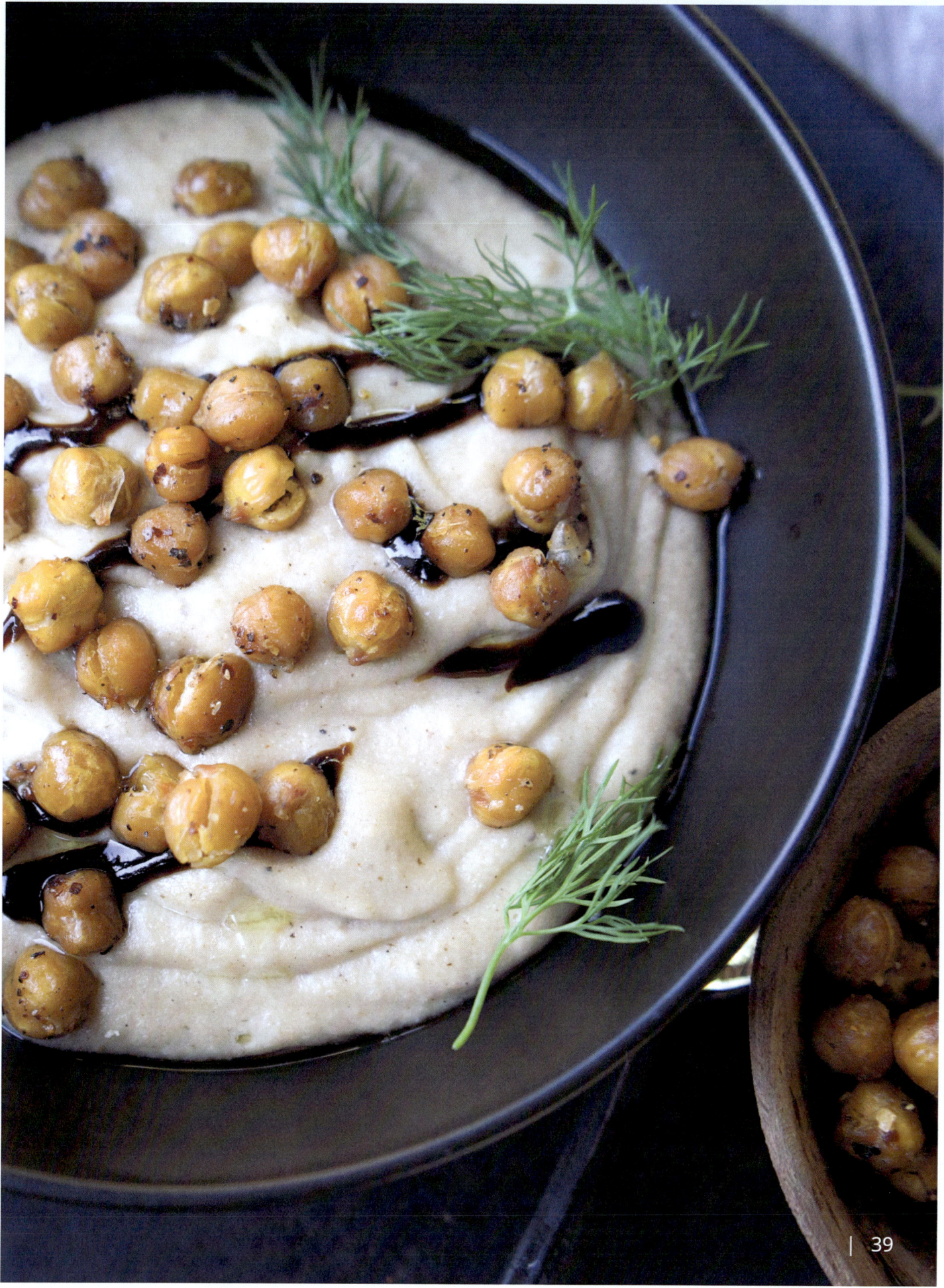

PUMPKIN LENTIL SOUP

When the weather cools down, this pumpkin lentil soup is the ultimate comfort meal—hearty, creamy, and packed with protein. Sure, you could roast a fresh pumpkin, but let's be real—canned pumpkin is a lifesaver. This version is fast, nutritious, and perfect for a weeknight dinner.

Ingredients

- **1 onion, chopped**
- **4 cloves garlic, minced**
- **2 cups mushrooms, chopped**
- **1 ½ cups carrots, shredded**
- **1 tbsp curry paste**
- **1 can (29 oz) pumpkin puree**
- **1 cup red lentils**
- **1 can (13.5 oz) coconut milk**
- **1 cup chicken broth**
- **Juice of 1 lime**
- **1 tbsp ginger paste**
- **1 tsp allspice**
- **1 tsp cinnamon powder**
- **Salt & pepper to taste**
- **Oil for sautéing**

Optional Protein Boosters:

- **1 can (15 oz) chickpeas**
- **1-2 cups shredded cooked chicken or turkey**
- **½ cup Greek yogurt (stirred in after cooking)**

Instructions

- Sauté: set Instant Pot to Sauté mode. Heat oil and cook onions until softened. Add garlic, mushrooms, and carrots; cook until tender.
- Pressure cook: add all remaining ingredients, stir, and seal the lid. Cook on Manual High Pressure for 10 minutes. Allow a natural release for 5 minutes, then quick release.
- Blend & serve: blend to desired consistency using an immersion blender. Adjust seasoning if needed.
- Add more protein: stir in your choice of protein boosters before serving.
- Top it off: serve with lime wedges, parsley, Greek yogurt, balsamic glaze, roasted pine nuts, or sautéed mushrooms.

Scan to watch

Serves 4

Prep time 5 min

Cook time 20 min

Quick Tips:
- Roast canned chickpeas with olive oil and spices at 400°F for 15 minutes for a crunchy topping.
- Freeze in portions for easy meal prep. Just reheat and serve!

Calories: 330 | Protein: 12g (boostable to 20-25g) | Carbs: 40g | Fat: 14g

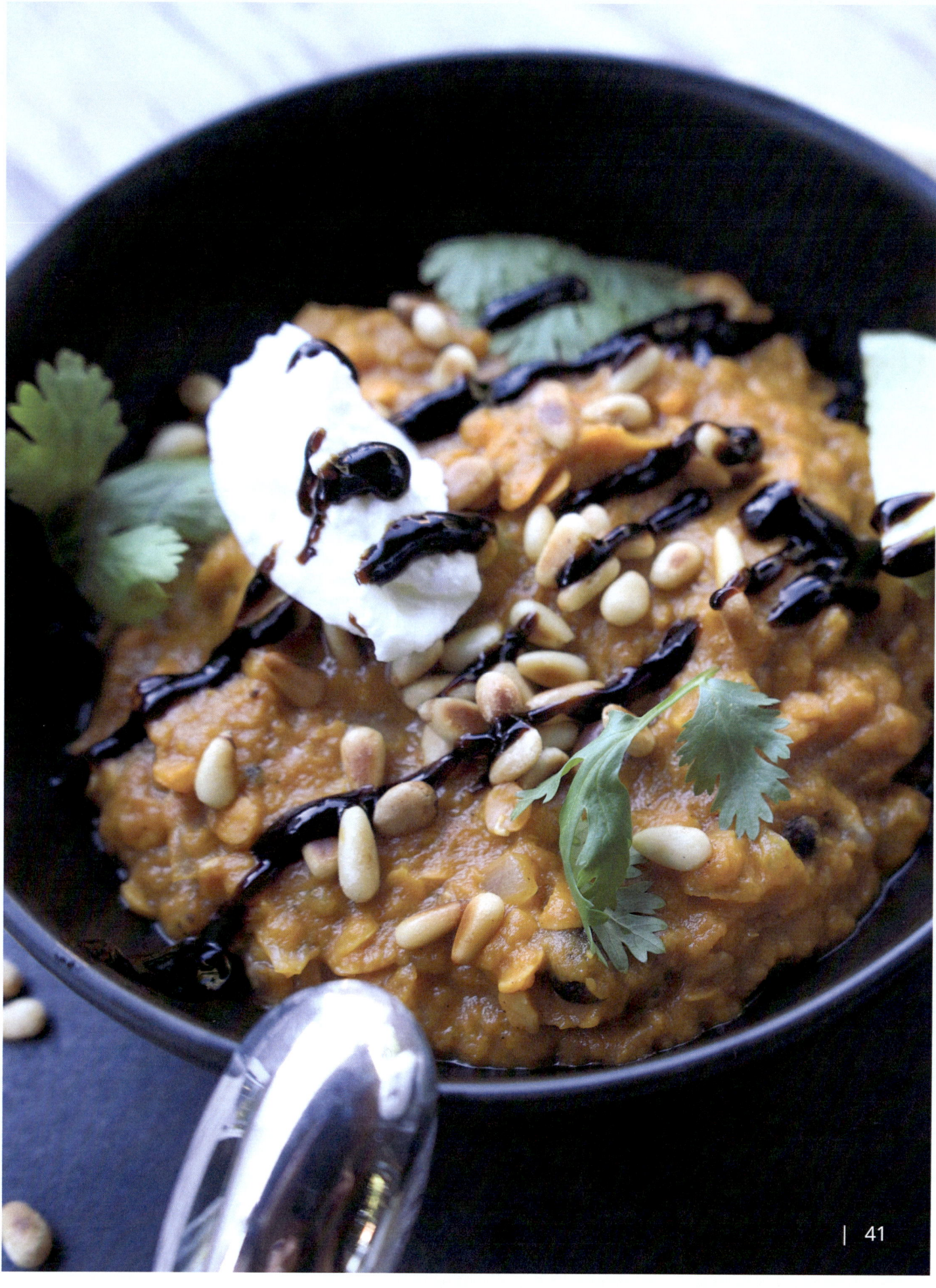

BUTTERNUT SQUASH LENTIL SOUP

When fall hits, it's time for roasted everything. This soup is like a warm hug—rich, creamy, and packed with protein thanks to lentils. Plus, it's secretly fancy without any extra effort. Perfect for a weeknight meal that tastes like you spent hours in the kitchen.

Ingredients

- **1 whole butternut squash (stab with a fork, microwave for 10 minutes)**
- **½ onion, chopped**
- **½ apple, chopped**
- **1 whole head garlic (cut top off for roasting)**
- **1 carrot, chopped**
- **1 cup cherry tomatoes**
- **1 bell pepper, chopped**
- **1 tsp salt**
- **½ tsp pepper**
- **½ tsp paprika**
- **½ tsp cumin**
- **2 tbsp olive oil**
- **1 tbsp fruit vinegar (apple cider or similar)**
- **1-2 sprigs fresh rosemary**
- **1 cup chicken broth**
- **1 can (14 oz) coconut milk**
- **1 cup red lentils**
- **Juice of 1 lime**

Instructions

- Poke holes in the squash with a fork and microwave for 10 minutes to soften. Slice in half.
- Place squash halves, onion, apple, garlic, carrot, cherry tomatoes, and bell pepper on a baking sheet. Season with salt, pepper, paprika, and cumin. Drizzle with olive oil and vinegar. Add rosemary sprigs. Roast at 425°F for 20-30 minutes until golden and tender.
- Scoop out the butternut squash flesh and blend with the roasted veggies and 1 cup of broth until smooth.
- Pour the blended mixture into a pot, stir in coconut milk and lentils. Simmer for 15 minutes, stirring occasionally. Add lime juice and adjust seasoning.
- Ladle into bowls, top with fried mushrooms, balsamic glaze, and parsley. Serve with lime wedges.

Scan to watch

Serves 5

Prep time 10 min

Cook time 45 min

Quick Tips:
- Time-Saver? Microwave squash first—it makes chopping a breeze.
- More Protein? Add shredded chicken, tofu or more lentils
- Make It Creamier? Blend in some Greek yogurt before serving.

Calories: 350 | Protein: 12g | Carbs: 40g | Fat: 18g

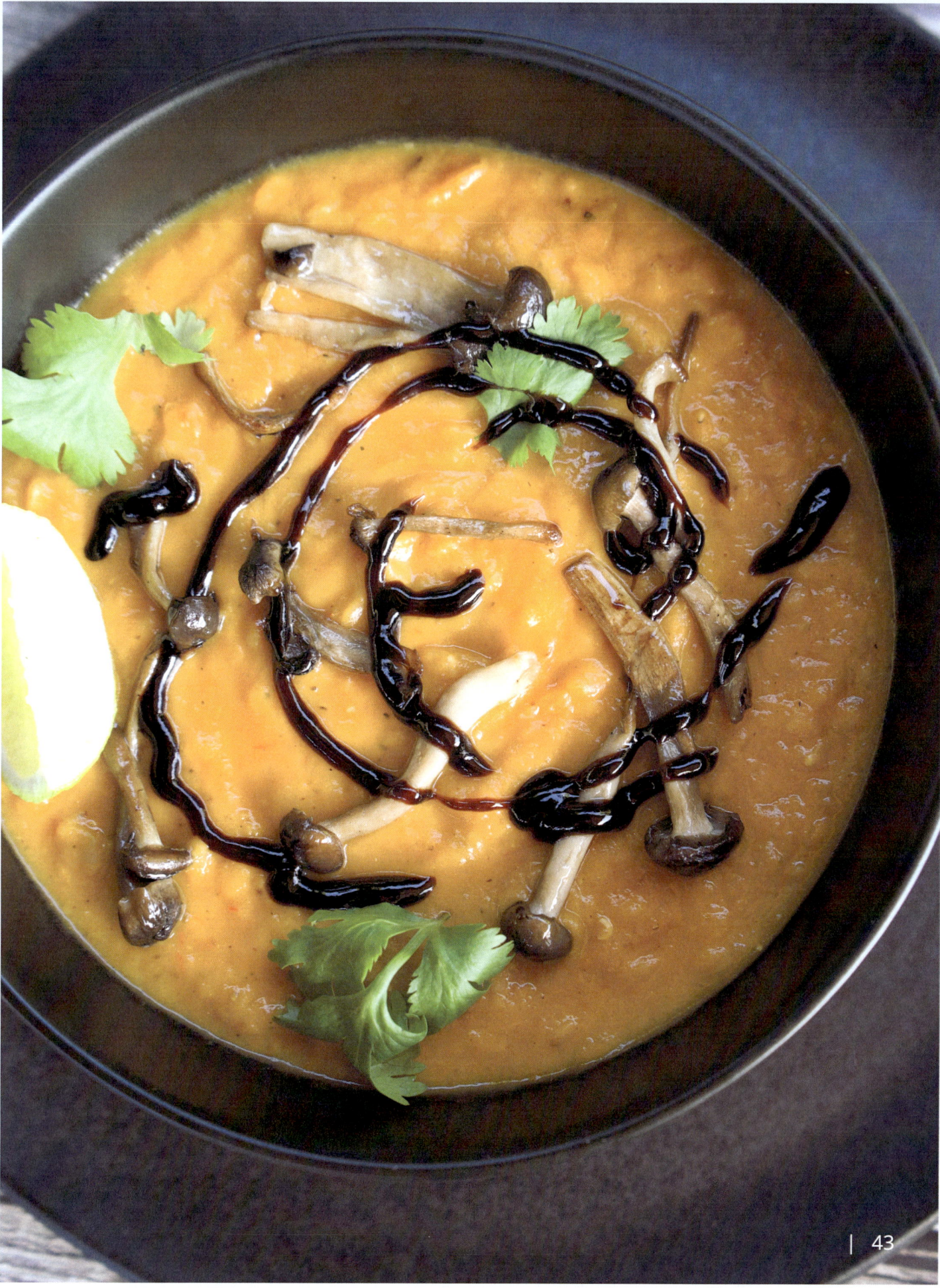

CAULIFLOWER LEEK SOUP

Minimal prep. Maximum comfort. My official favorite soup of the season—ready in under 30 minutes and fully customizable.

Ingredients

- **2 leeks — thinly sliced**
- **4 cloves garlic — minced**
- **Oil — for sautéing**
- **1 head cauliflower — chopped**
- **1 ½ tbsp butter chicken seasoning (or curry powder)**
- **Salt, pepper, chili flakes — to taste**
- **4 cups chicken broth**
- **Hot water — as needed for desired consistency**
- **1 lemon — juiced**
- **1 ½ cups Greek yogurt**

Optional Toppings:
- **Grilled cheese croutons**
- **Grilled thyme**
- **Extra virgin olive oil**
- **Balsamic glaze**

Instructions

- Sauté: heat oil in a large pot. Add leeks and garlic; cook until soft and fragrant, about 5 minutes. Add cauliflower and cook another few minutes. Stir in seasoning, salt, pepper, and chili flakes.
- Broth: pour in broth and enough hot water to just cover the veggies. Bring to a boil, then simmer until cauliflower is fork-tender (15–20 minutes).
- Blend: stir in Greek yogurt and lemon juice. Blend until silky smooth using an immersion blender.
- Top it off: pour into bowls and get creative—grilled cheese croutons, thyme, a drizzle of olive oil, or balsamic glaze.

Scan to watch

Serves 4

Prep time 10 min

Cook time 20 min

Quick Tips:
- This cozy bowl freezes beautifully for future lazy days.
- Customize the thickness by adjusting the hot water.

Calories: ~180 | Protein: ~10g | Carbs: ~14g | Fat: ~10g

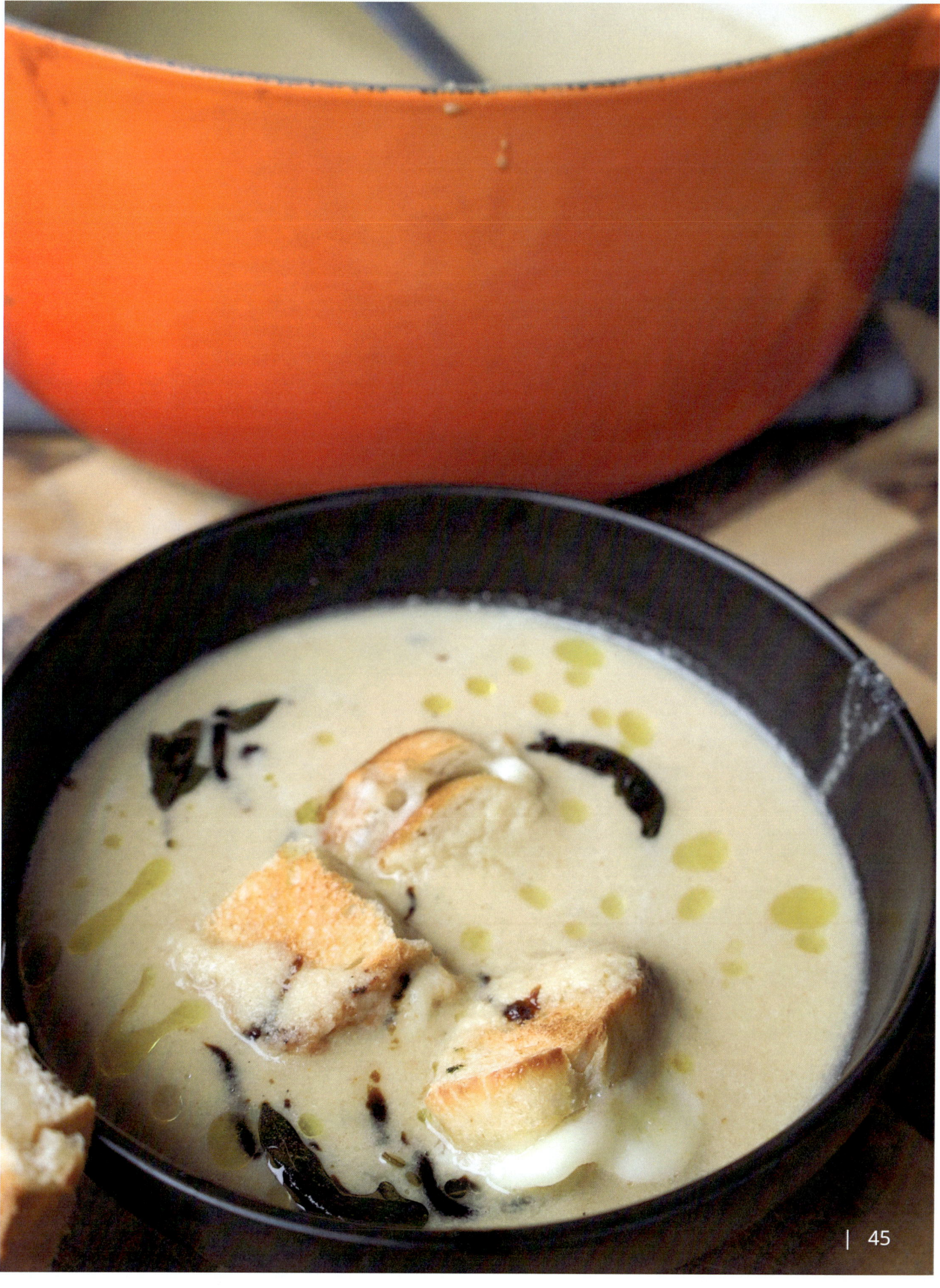

TURKEY TORTILLA SOUP

Leftover turkey looking like a crime scene in the fridge? Let's fix that. This colorful, cozy soup transforms sad scraps (and even the carcass) into a bowl of post-holiday greatness. Thanks to the Instant Pot, it's ready in 30 minutes—fast enough for your food-coma recovery mission.

Ingredients

- **1 onion — chopped**
- **3 garlic cloves — minced**
- **2 bell peppers — chopped**
- **1 (14 oz) can black beans — drained and rinsed**
- **1 cup frozen corn**
- **2 cups cooked turkey — chopped**
- **1 turkey carcass — optional but highly recommended**
- **1 (14 oz) can diced tomatoes**
- **3 tbsp tomato paste**
- **Juice of 1 lime**
- **4 cups chicken broth**
- **Spices: 1 tsp paprika, 1 tsp cumin, 1 tsp chili powder, salt & pepper**
- **Oil — for sautéing**
- *Toppings: lime wedges, jalapeño slices, cilantro, sour cream, tortilla chips, shredded cheese, avocado.*

Instructions

- Set Instant Pot to "Sauté." Add oil, then cook onion and garlic for 3 minutes. Toss in bell peppers and cook 2 more minutes.
- Add paprika, cumin, chili powder, salt, and pepper. Stir for 30 seconds to wake up those spices.
- Add black beans, corn, diced tomatoes, and tomato paste. Stir everything together.
- Mix in chopped turkey and turkey carcass. Pour in chicken broth and give it a good stir.
- Close the lid. Pressure Cook (Manual) for 10 minutes. Quick release when done.
- Remove carcass. Stir in lime juice and adjust seasoning to taste.

Scan to watch

Serves 4

Prep time 10 min

Cook time 20 min

Quick Tips:
- No Instant Pot? Simmer everything in a regular pot for 25 minutes.
- Serve hot and pile on your favorites—cilantro, sour cream, cheese, chips, avocado—go wild.

Calories: ~350 | Protein: ~28g | Carbs: ~30g | Fat: ~14g

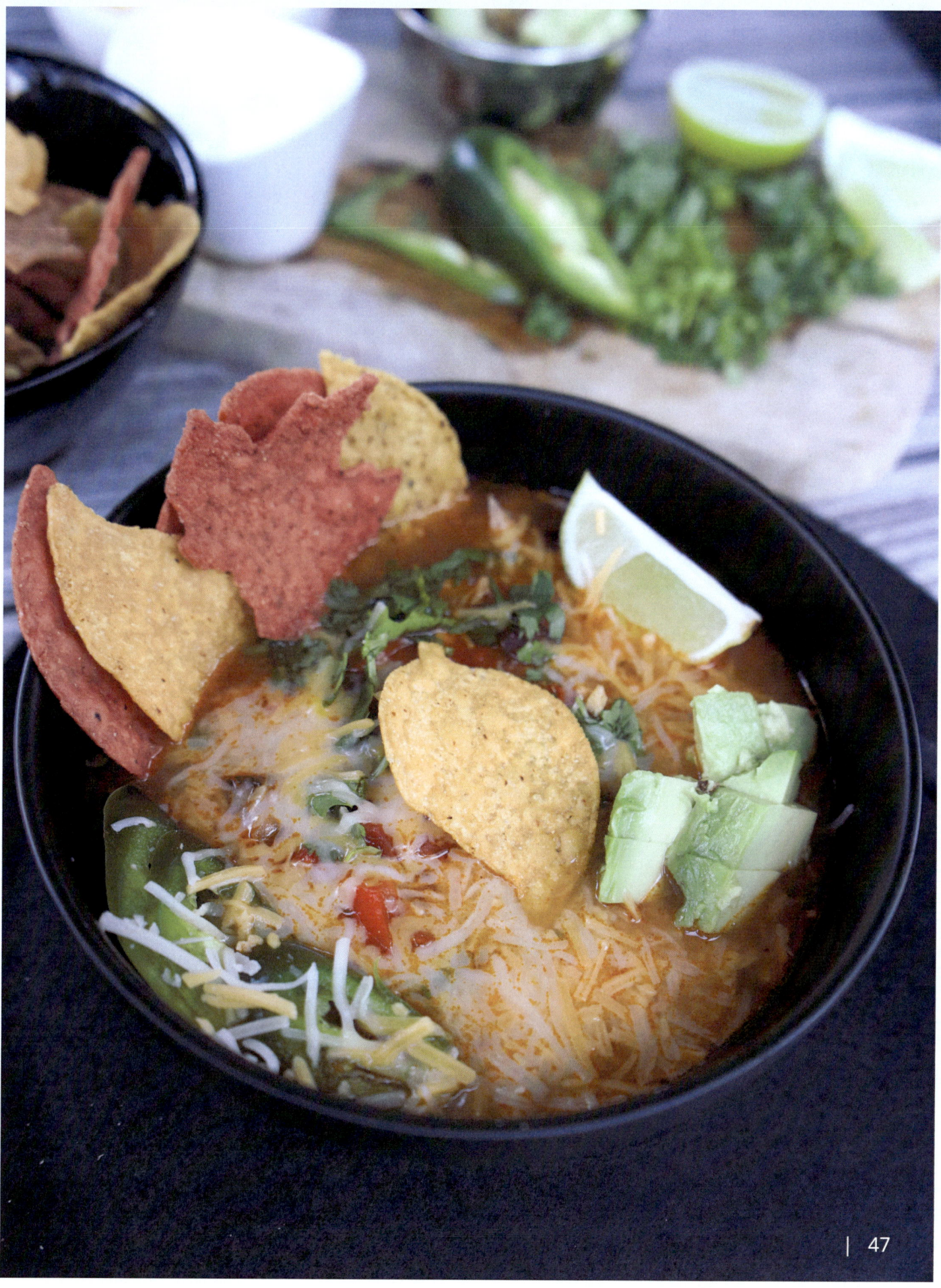

COCONUT FISH CURRY WITH LIME & LEMONGRASS

After throwing down over 100 new dishes this year, this Coconut Fish Curry stole the crown. Bold, aromatic, and impossible to get tired of, it's packed with the lush flavors of lemongrass, lime, and creamy coconut milk. Think: comfort food, but make it tropical and protein-packed.

Ingredients

- **4 white fish filets (cod, tilapia, or snapper) — cut into chunks**
- **3 tbsp lime juice**
- **Salt — to taste**
- **2 tbsp vegetable oil**
- **1 onion — finely chopped**
- **3 garlic cloves — minced**
- **1-inch piece of ginger — grated**
- **2 stalks lemongrass — bruised and cut into 2-inch pieces**
- **3 Thai red chilies**
- **2 tsp turmeric powder**
- **2 tsp ground coriander**
- **2 (14 oz) cans coconut milk**
- **1 tbsp fish sauce**
- **2 tsp sugar**
- **5 kaffir lime leaves**
- **Zest and juice of 1 lime**
- **1 tbsp red curry paste**

Instructions

- Marinate fish chunks with lime juice and salt; set aside for 10 minutes.
- Heat oil in a skillet. Sauté onion 3–4 minutes, add garlic, ginger, and lemongrass, cooking another 1–2 minutes. Stir in chilies, turmeric, and coriander.
- Pour in coconut milk, add fish sauce, sugar, kaffir lime leaves, lime zest, and red curry paste. Bring to a simmer.
- Add marinated fish to the curry. Cover and simmer 10 minutes, until the fish is cooked through.
- Remove from heat, stir in lime juice. Taste and adjust seasoning if needed.
- Ladle into bowls, garnish with cilantro, Thai basil, red chilies, and lime wedges. Serve hot with coconut rice.

Scan to watch

Serves 4

Prep time 15 min

Cook time 20 min

Quick Tips:
- Lemongrass tip: smash the stalks for maximum flavor release.
- Fish swap: salmon or shrimp also work—just watch the cooking time.

Calories: ~450 | Protein: ~38g | Carbs: ~18g | Fat: ~28g

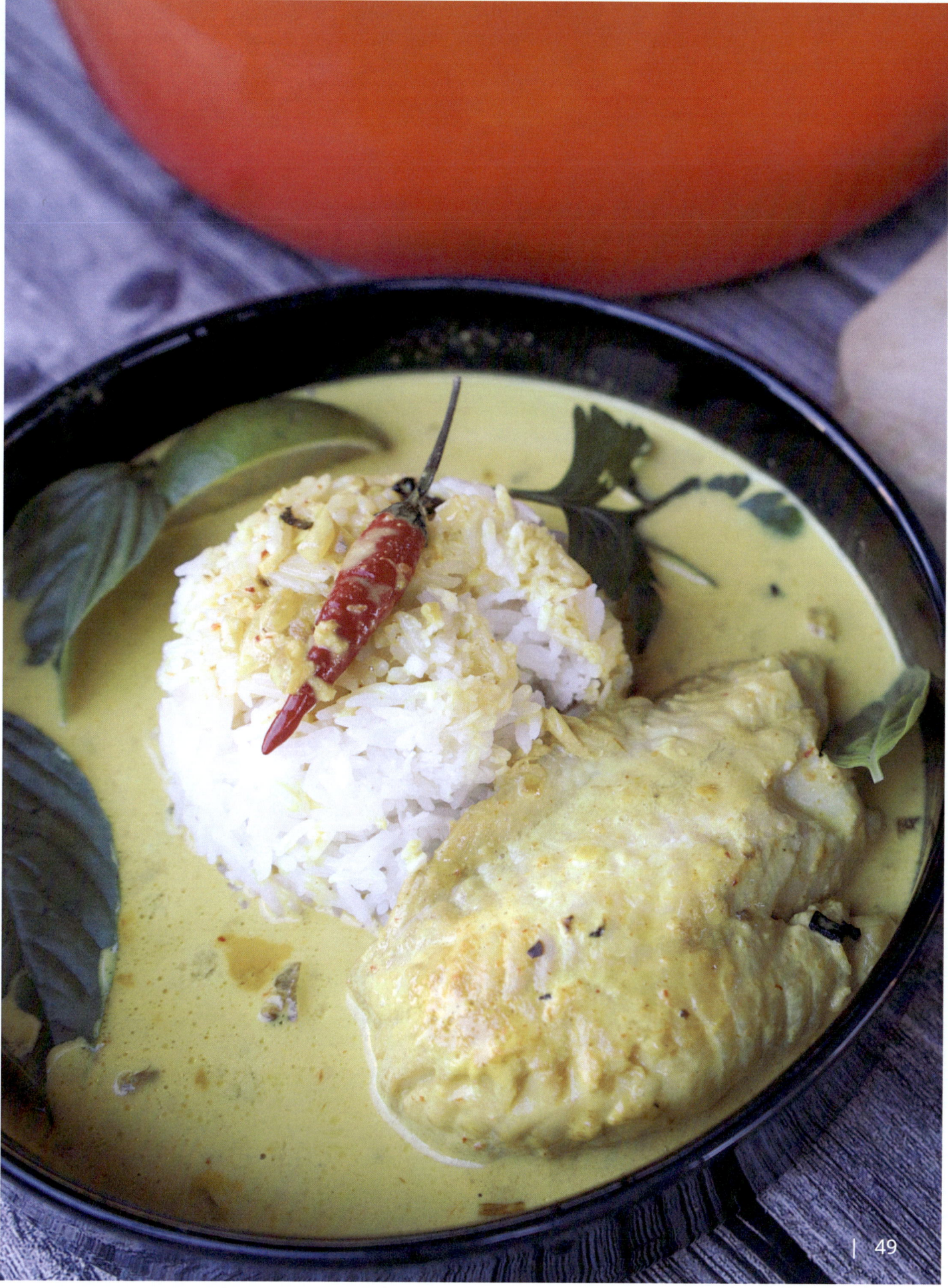

INSTANT POT BEEF BOURGUIGNON

Classic French comfort food—minus the all-day cooking drama. This Instant Pot version gives you deep, slow-simmered flavor in under an hour. Think rich wine sauce, melt-in-your-mouth beef, and pearl onions so good you'll eat them first.

Ingredients

- **2.5 lbs beef chuck, cut into 1.5-inch cubes**
- **6 slices bacon, chopped**
- **3 cups pearl onions (frozen or fresh, peeled)**
- **2 carrots, thickly sliced**
- **1 onion, chopped**
- **5 cloves garlic, minced**
- **4 cups sliced mushrooms**
- **2 cups dry red wine (Burgundy or Pinot Noir)**
- **2 cups beef broth**
- **2 tbsp tomato paste**
- **2 tbsp flour (or cornstarch for gluten-free)**
- **1 tbsp olive oil**
- **1 tbsp soy sauce**
- **3 sprigs fresh thyme (or 2 tsp dried)**
- **1 bay leaf**
- **Salt and pepper to taste**

Instructions

- Set Instant Pot to sauté. Cook bacon until crispy; remove and set aside.
- Season beef with salt and pepper. Sear in batches until browned; remove and set aside with bacon.
- Sauté chopped onion, carrots, and pearl onions for 5 minutes until golden. Add garlic and cook 1 minute.
- Stir in tomato paste and flour; cook 1 minute. Pour in wine, scrape up browned bits, and simmer 2 minutes.
- Return beef, bacon, and mushrooms to pot. Add broth, soy sauce, thyme, and bay leaf. Stir to combine.
- Seal lid. Pressure cook on high for 35 minutes. Natural release for 10 minutes, then quick-release.
- Taste and adjust seasoning. To thicken, simmer on sauté mode until sauce reduces.

Scan to watch

Serves 4

Prep time 20 min

Cook time 55 min

Quick Tips:
- For crispier bacon place bacon in a cold Instant Pot, then set to sauté.
- Serve with egg noodles, mashed potatoes, crusty bread, or cauliflower mash for a low-carb option.

Cal: 400 with cauliflower mash|Protein: 40g|Carbs:14g|Fat: 20g

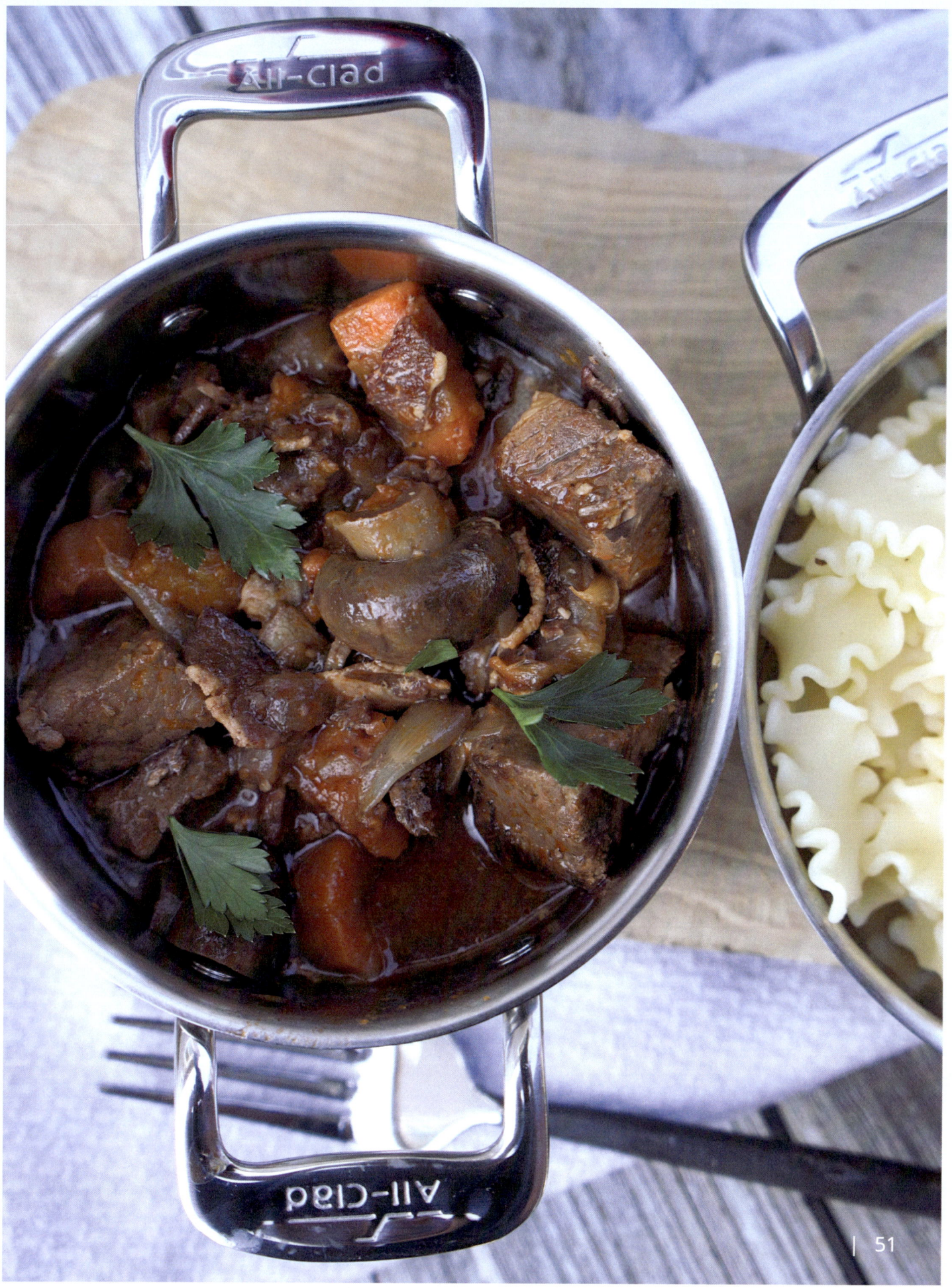

INSTANT POT PASTA FAGIOLI SOUP

A protein-packed twist on the Italian classic—this soup's got 2 pounds of meat, beans, pasta, and serious flavor. It tastes like it simmered all day but comes together in 30 minutes, thanks to the Instant Pot.

Ingredients

- **2 lb ground meat (beef, turkey, or chicken)**
- **2 tbsp olive oil**
- **1 medium onion, chopped**
- **5 garlic cloves, minced**
- **2 carrots, diced**
- **2 celery stalks, diced**
- **1 (14 oz) can diced tomatoes**
- **1 (14 oz) can San Marzano tomatoes**
- **1 (14 oz) can white beans, rinsed and drained**
- **1 (14 oz) can butter beans, rinsed and drained**
- **6 cups chicken broth**
- **2 cups small dried pasta**
- **3 tbsp tomato paste**
- **1 tsp dried oregano**
- **1 tsp dried basil**
- **2 bay leaves**
- **Salt and pepper to taste**
- **For garnish: Parmesan cheese, parsley or basil**

Instructions

- Sauté the aromatics: set Instant Pot to sauté mode. Heat olive oil, then cook onion, garlic, carrots, and celery for 3–4 minutes.
- Brown the meat: add ground meat, break it up, cook until browned, and season with salt and pepper.
- Build the base: stir in tomato paste, oregano, basil, bay leaves, tomatoes, and broth. Mix well.
- Pressure cook: seal the lid and cook on high for 10 minutes. Natural release for 5 minutes, then quick release.
- Add pasta and beans: set to sauté. Stir in pasta and beans. Simmer for 10 minutes or until pasta is tender.
- Serve: ladle into bowls, top with Parmesan and herbs.

Scan to watch

Serves 6

Prep time 10 min

Cook time 20 min

Quick Tips:
- Skip the Instant Pot? Use a stovetop pot and simmer 25–30 minutes before adding pasta and beans.
- Skip pasta in leftovers to avoid sogginess—add fresh when reheating.

Calories: ~320 | Protein: ~28g | Carbs: ~30g | Fat: ~12g

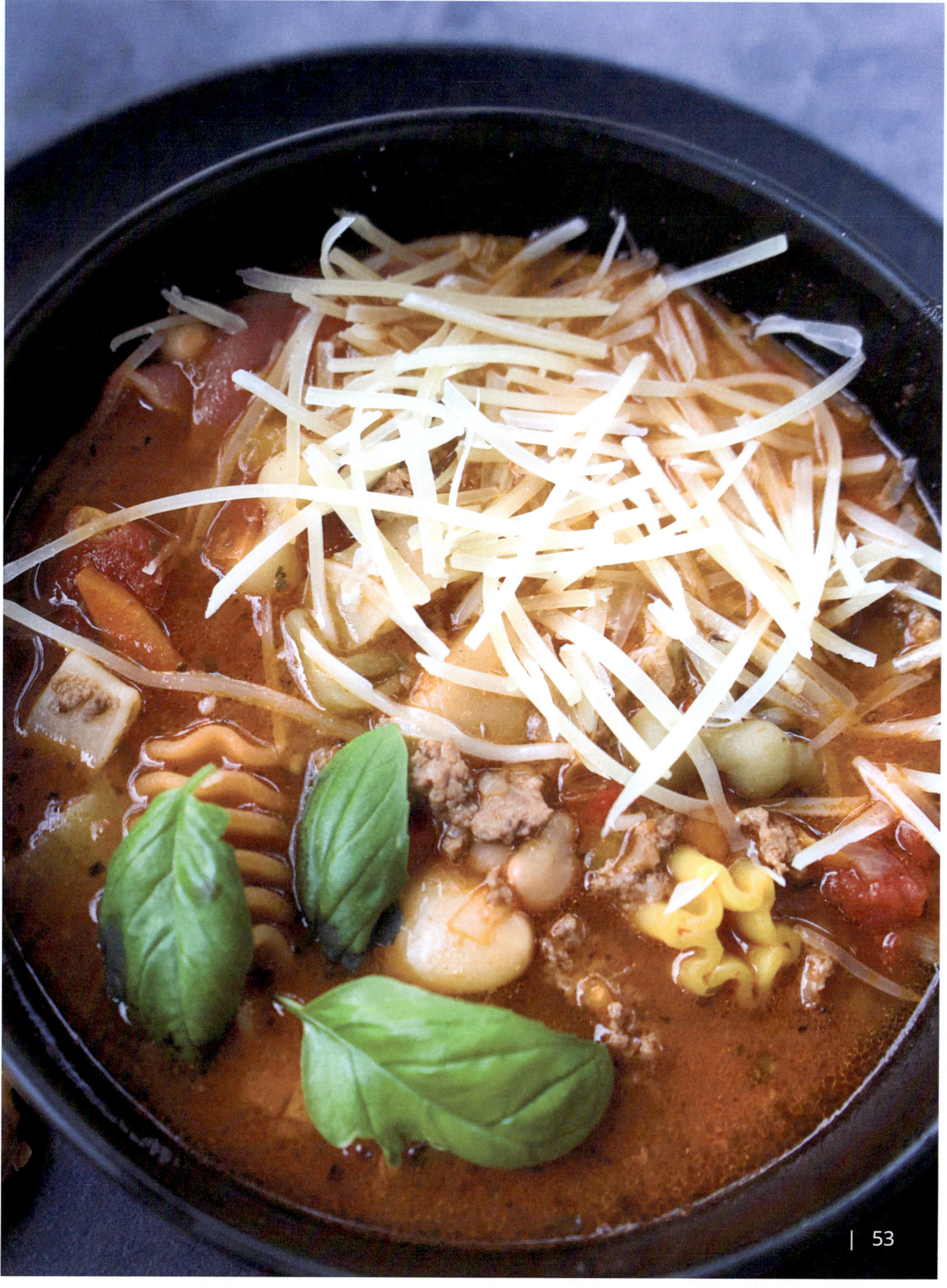

INSTANT POT CHICKEN LEMON SOUP

Creamy, zesty, and pure comfort—this soup gives you cozy vibes without wrecking your macros. Lean chicken, veggies, and a Greek yogurt twist make this a weeknight winner.

Ingredients

- **2 tbsp olive oil**
- **2 lb chicken (breast or thighs), cut in chunks**
- **1 medium onion, chopped**
- **4 garlic cloves, minced**
- **2 large carrots, diced**
- **6 cups low-sodium chicken broth**
- **1 cup quinoa or orzo (optional)**
- **½ cup plain Greek yogurt**
- **3 tbsp lemon juice**
- **1 tsp lemon zest**
- **1 tsp dried oregano**
- **1–2 sprigs rosemary**
- **1–2 bay leaves**
- **½ tsp cumin (optional)**
- **½ tsp turmeric**
- **Salt & pepper to taste**
- **Fresh parsley or dill (garnish)**

Instructions

- Sauté the chicken: set Instant Pot to Sauté. Heat oil, brown chicken for 3–4 mins. Remove and set aside.
- Cook the veggies: add onion, garlic, carrots. Sauté 3–4 mins, scraping up bits.
- Build the base: return chicken. Add broth, herbs, spices, and quinoa/orzo if using. Season lightly.
- Pressure cook: seal lid. Cook on high pressure for 10 mins. Quick release.
- Cream it up: whisk yogurt, lemon juice, and zest in a bowl. Temper with hot soup. Stir into pot slowly—don't boil.
- Taste & serve: adjust lemon, salt, and pepper. Garnish with parsley or dill. Serve warm.

Scan to watch

Serves 4

Prep time 10 min

Cook time 15 min

Quick Tips:
- No curdle zone: Always temper the yogurt first.
- Want it grain-free? Skip quinoa/orzo—still filling.
- Instant Pot hack: frozen chicken works—just add 2 mins to pressure time.

Calories: ~280 (no grains) | Protein: ~40g | Carbs: ~8g (more with grains) | Fat: ~8g

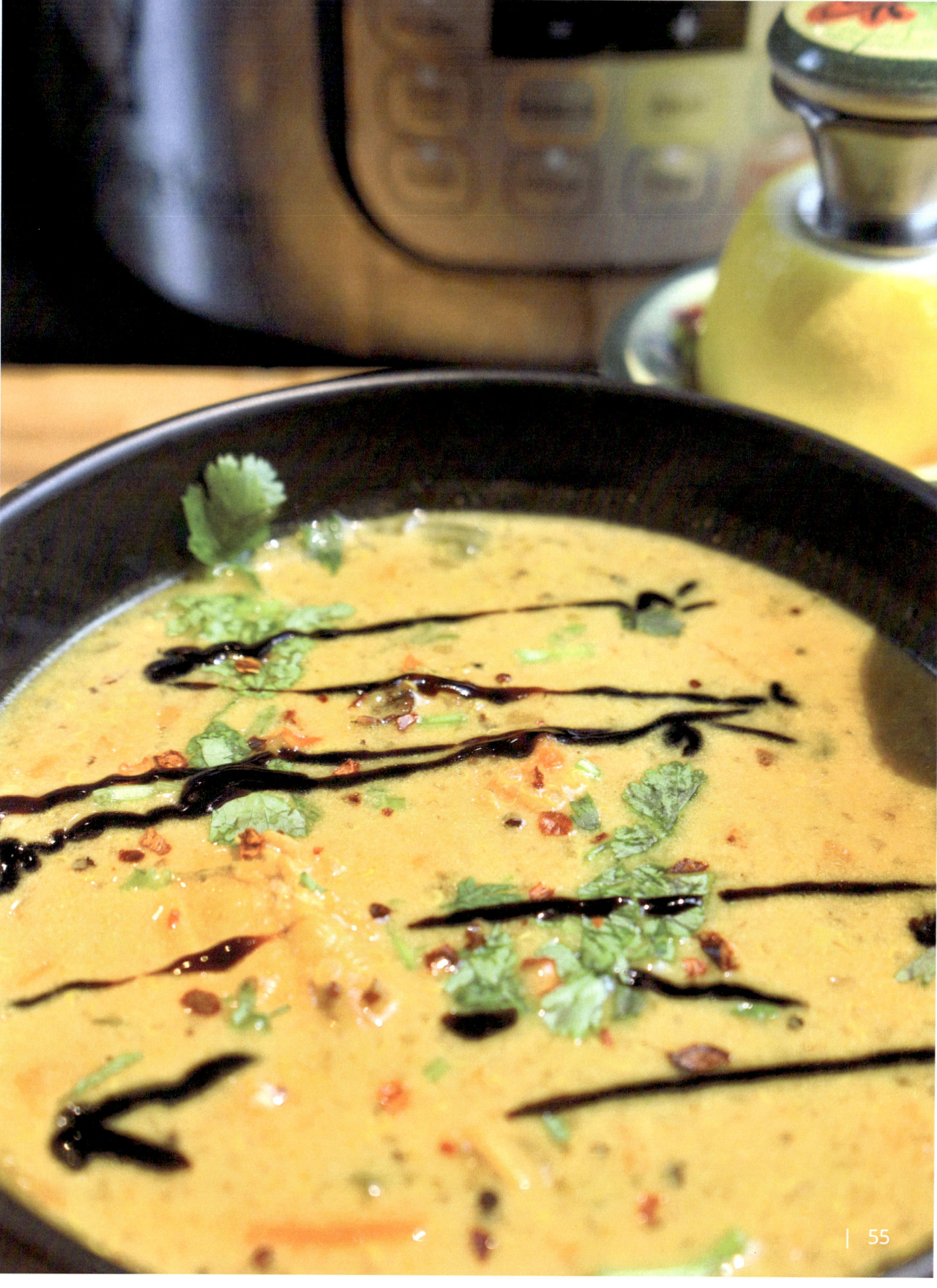

HIGH-PROTEIN THAI RED CURRY NOODLE SOUP WITH CRISPY GYOZAS

This spicy, creamy noodle soup delivers all the bold flavors of a Thai curry. Juicy chicken, aromatic herbs, silky coconut broth, and crispy gyozas on top for that "did I really make this?" moment. One pot, one Instant Pot.

Ingredients

- **1 tbsp coconut oil**
- **1 shallot, chopped**
- **1 carrot, chopped**
- **4 cloves garlic, chopped**
- **2 tsp fresh ginger, minced**
- **1 tbsp Thai red curry paste**
- **3 cups mushrooms, sliced**
- **1 can (19 oz) coconut milk**
- **4 cups chicken stock**
- **Juice of 1 lime**
- **2 stalks lemongrass**
- **3 kaffir lime leaves (tied in cheesecloth or a tea bag)**
- **1 tbsp fish sauce**
- **3–4 boneless, skinless chicken thighs**
- **Rice noodles, cooked according to package**
- **12 gyozas, fried (follow package instructions)**
- **Handful of Thai basil leaves, for garnish**

Instructions

- Set Instant Pot to sauté. Heat coconut oil, then add shallot, carrot, garlic, and ginger. Cook 2 minutes.
- Stir in red curry paste. Add mushrooms and sauté for another 2 minutes.
- Pour in chicken stock and coconut milk. Add lime juice, bruised lemongrass, fish sauce, and the leaf bundle.
- Add chicken thighs. Seal the lid and pressure cook on high for 10 min.
- Boil rice noodles and fry gyozas.
- Quick release the pressure. Remove leaf bundles. Shred chicken and return it to the pot.
- Add noodles to bowls, ladle in hot soup, and top with crispy gyozas and Thai basil. Serve with lime wedges.

Scan to watch

Serves 6

Prep time 10 min

Cook time 20 min

Quick Tips:
- Want to meal-prep? Store broth and noodles separately to avoid soggy noodles. Reheat and combine when serving.
- No Instant Pot? Simmer everything on the stovetop for 25–30 minutes, partially covered.

Calories: 450 | Protein: 28g | Carbs: 42g | Fat: 18g

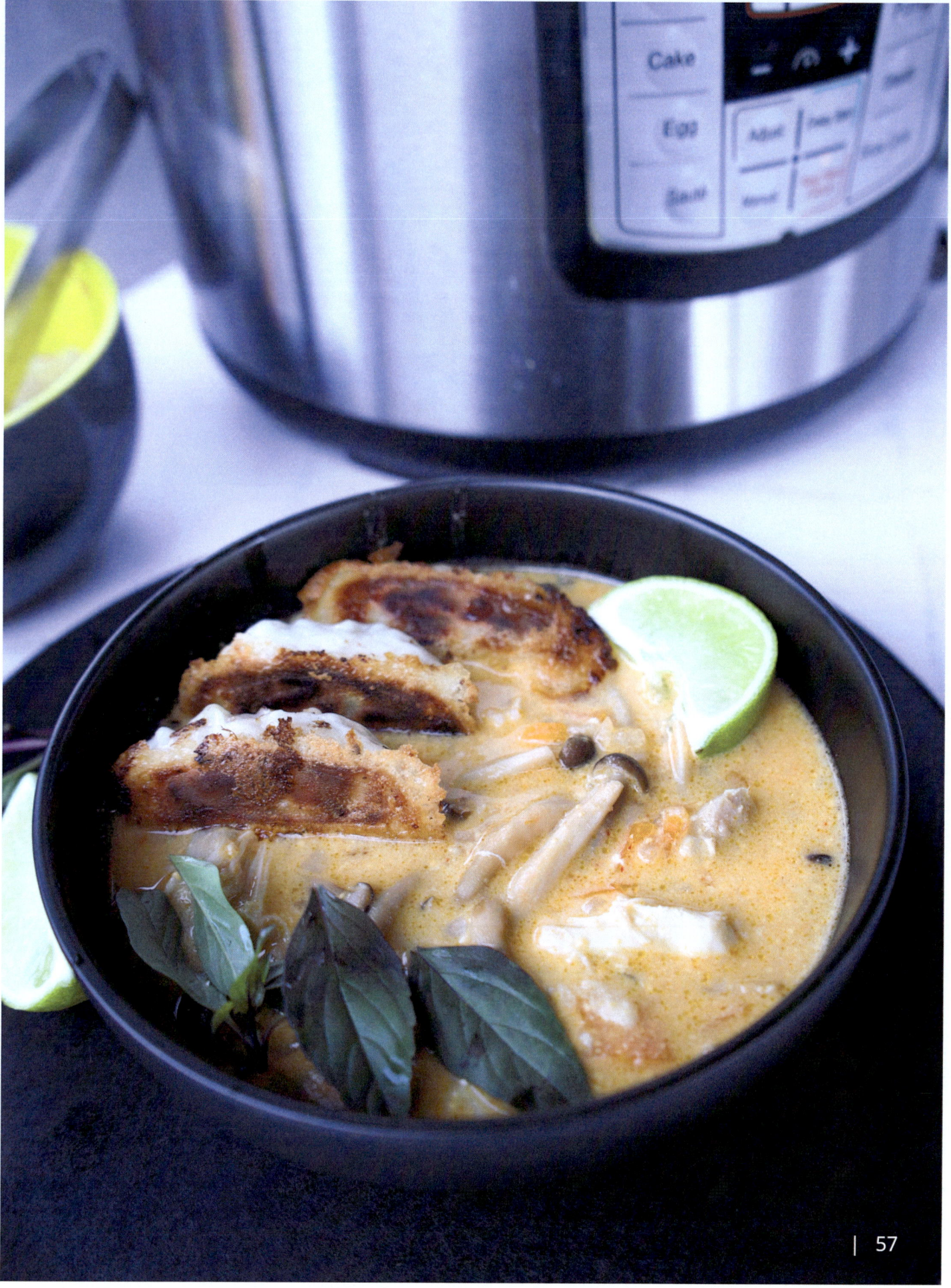

INSTANT POT CHICKEN PHO

Why pay for takeout when you can drop flavor bombs in your kitchen in 30 minutes flat? This deeply aromatic Vietnamese soup is warm, nourishing, and shockingly easy with a little Instant Pot magic.

Ingredients

For the Broth:
- 2 lb bone-in, chicken thighs
- 1 tbsp oil
- 2-inch fresh ginger – peeled and halved
- 1 onion – peeled and halved
- 6 cups chicken broth
- 4 sprigs parsley
- 1 tbsp fish sauce
- 1 tsp sugar
- 1 tsp salt (adjust to taste)
- 1 cinnamon stick
- 3 star anise
- 3 whole cloves

For Serving:
- 7 oz thin rice noodles
- 1 cup bean sprouts
- ¼ cup chopped scallions
- ¼ cup chopped cilantro
- 1 lime – cut into wedges
- 1 jalapeño – thinly sliced
- Thai basil, hoisin sauce, and sriracha

Instructions

- Char aromatics: sauté halved onion and ginger in Instant Pot (no oil) until charred, ~2 mins.
- Add broth ingredients: add oil, spices, chicken, broth, parsley, fish sauce, salt, and sugar.
- Pressure cook: manual (High) for 15 mins. Let pressure naturally release for 10, then quick-release.
- Shred chicken & strain broth: discard bones/skin. Strain out aromatics and spices.
- Cook noodles: prepare according to package instructions.
- Assemble bowls: layer noodles, shredded chicken, and broth.
- Garnish: add sprouts, herbs, scallions, lime, and optional sauces. Slurp immediately.

Scan to watch

Serves 4

Prep time 10 min

Cook time 20 min

Quick Tips:
- Low-carb swap: use shirataki noodles or skip noodles altogether.
- Protein boost: add more chicken or toss in boiled egg halves.
- No Instant Pot? Simmer on the stove for 45–60 mins until chicken is tender.

Calories: ~380 | Protein: ~35g | Carbs: ~45g | Fat: ~8g

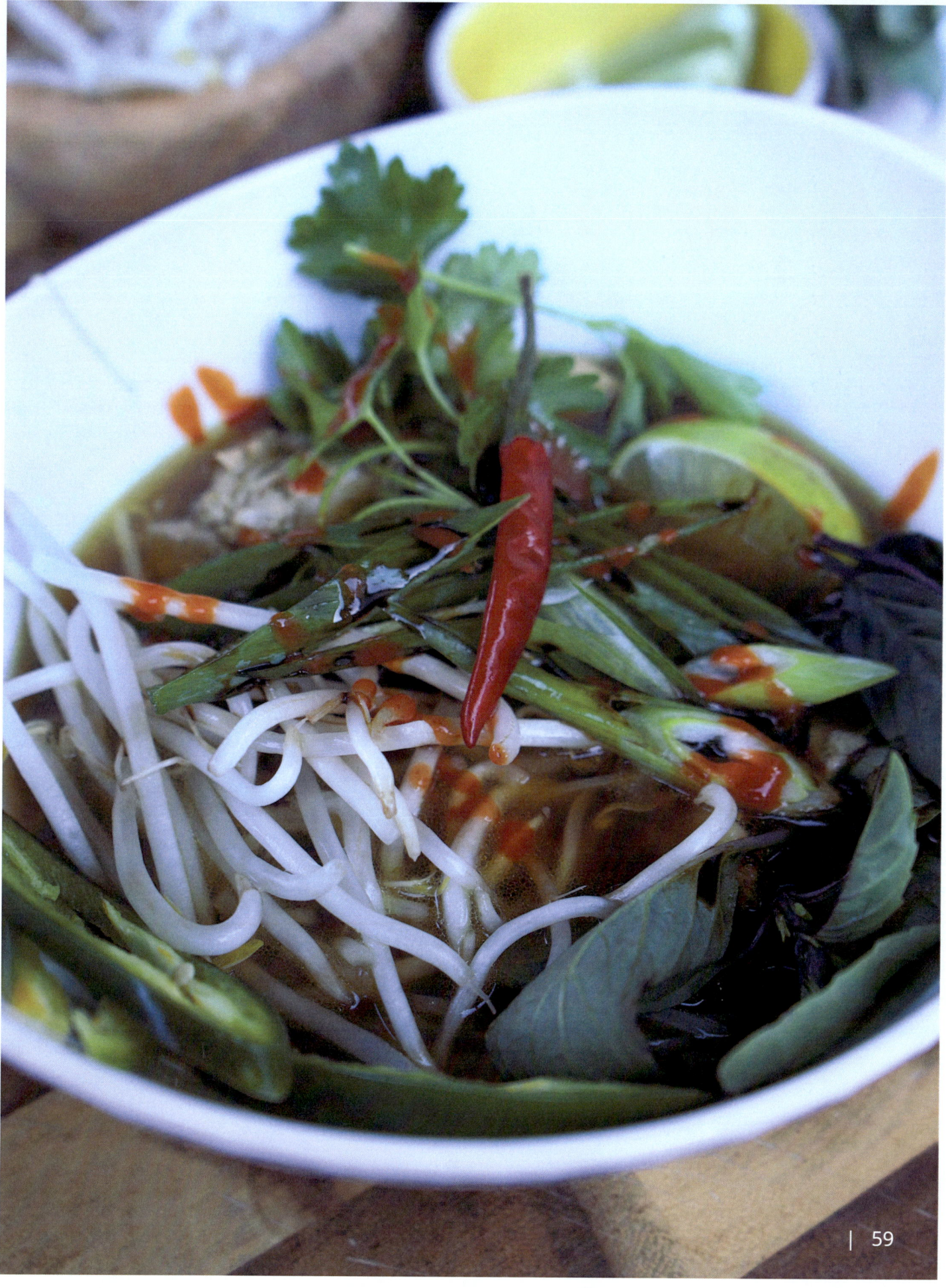

CARNE EN SU JUGO (MEXICAN BEEF STEW)

Whether you like it brothy like a soup or hearty like a stew, this high-protein, low-carb Mexican comfort classic hits the spot. The smoky, herby flavor comes together fast in the Instant Pot.

Ingredients

- **6 strips bacon, chopped**
- **2½ lbs flank steak, cubed**
- **6 tomatillos**
- **1 cup cilantro**
- **1 red onion, roughly chopped**
- **2 jalapeños, stems removed**
- **4 cloves garlic**
- **6 cups beef broth, divided**
- **Juice of 1 lime**
- **Salt & pepper, to taste**
- **½ tsp cumin**
- **½ tsp oregano**
- **2 cans (14 oz each) pinto beans, drained and rinsed**

Optional toppings: fried corn, chips, diced avocado, lime wedges, sliced jalapeños, chopped scallions and sour cream

Instructions

- Set Instant Pot to sauté. Fry the chopped bacon until crispy. Remove and set aside.
- In the same pot, add flank steak. Cook until browned. Season with salt and pepper. Turn off sauté.
- In a blender, combine tomatillos, cilantro, red onion, jalapeños, garlic, and ½ cup beef broth. Blend until smooth.
- Pour the sauce into the pot with the beef. Add remaining 5½ cups beef broth, lime juice, cumin, oregano, and the cooked bacon.
- Seal the lid and set to Manual – High Pressure for 10 minutes. Quick release the pressure.
- Turn sauté back on. Stir in pinto beans and cook for 4 minutes.

Scan to watch

Serves 8

Prep time
15 min

Cook time
25 min

Quick Tips:
- A rich, flavorful broth makes all the difference. Homemade or high-quality store-bought is worth it.
- Add more broth for a soupier vibe, or simmer uncovered a bit at the end for a thicker stew.

Calories: ~280 Protein: ~25g Carbs: ~12g Fat: ~15g

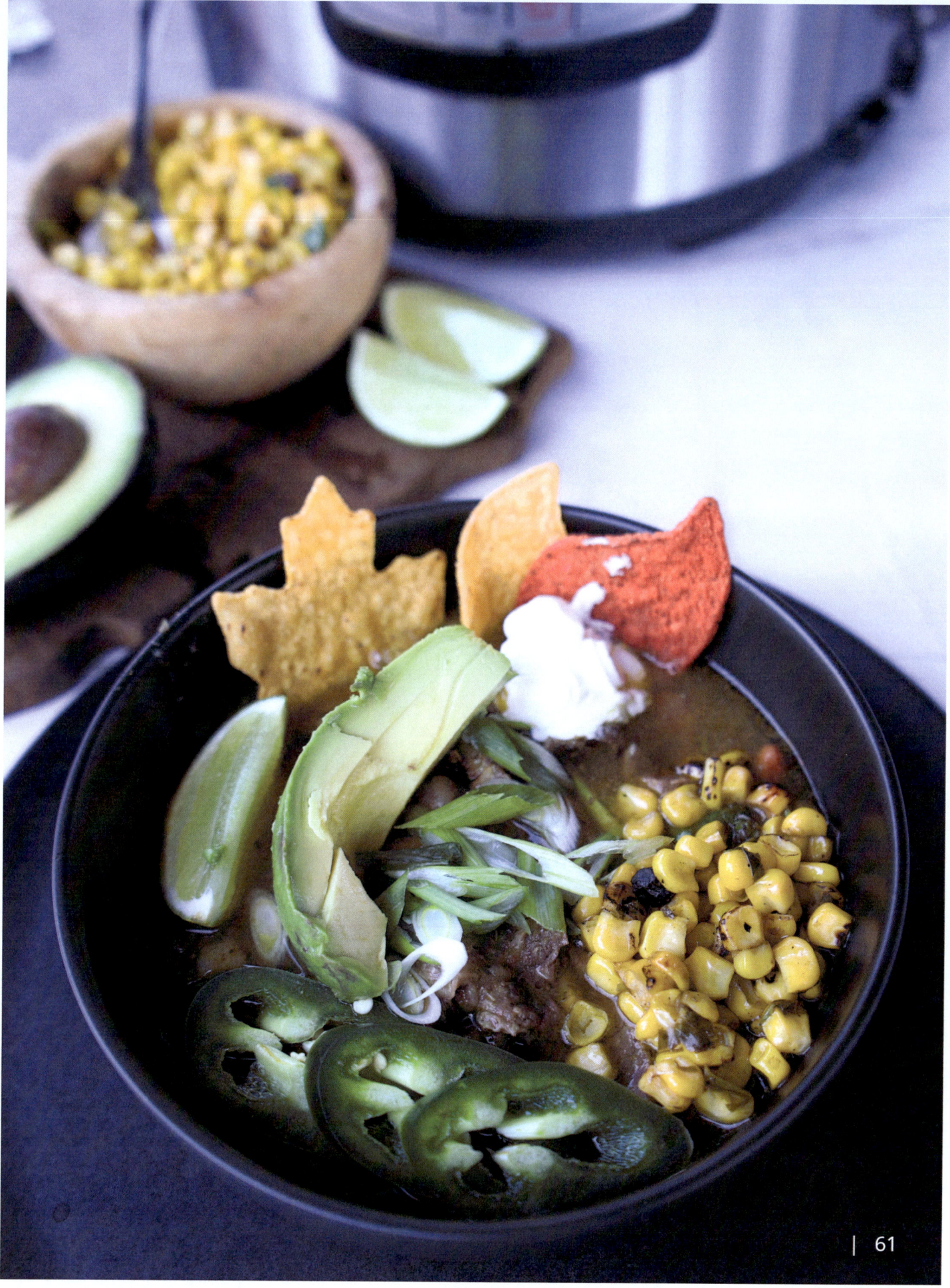

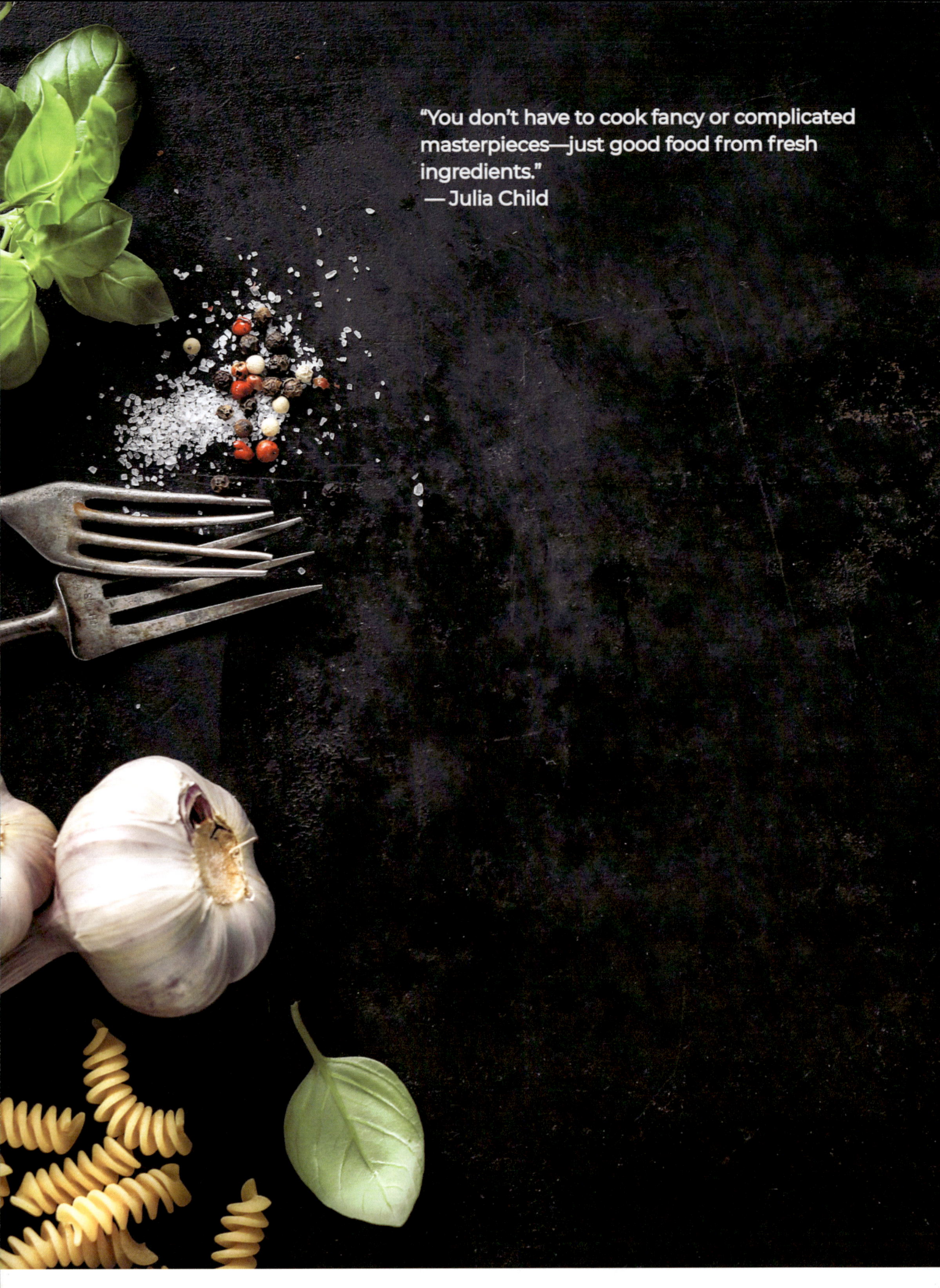

"You don't have to cook fancy or complicated masterpieces—just good food from fresh ingredients."
— Julia Child

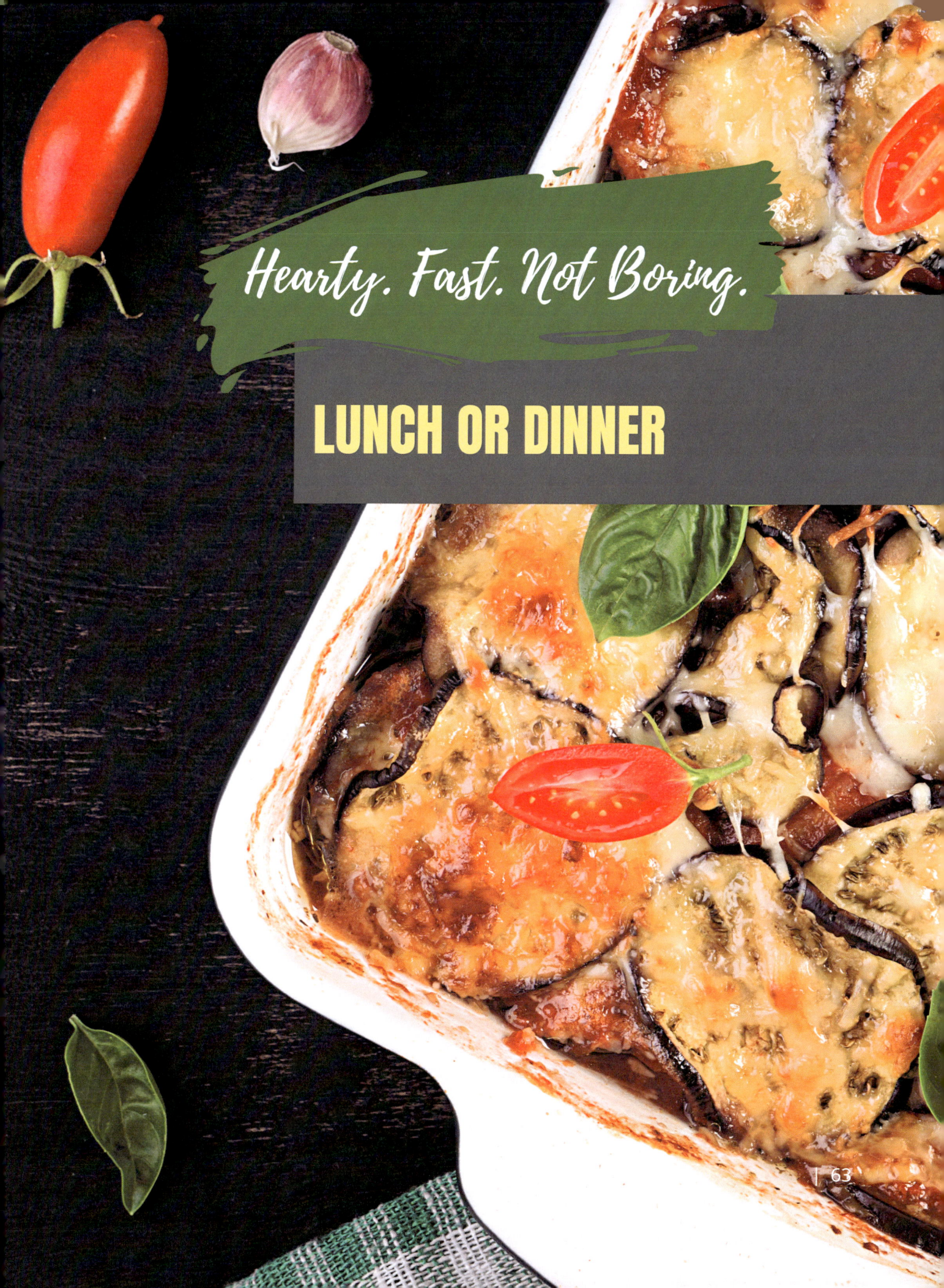

Hearty. Fast. Not Boring.
LUNCH OR DINNER

SMOKY AIR-FRIED LAMB CHOPS WITH MINT SAUCE AND PEACHES

Did you know you can make the best smoky lamb chops in the air fryer? Yep, fancy dinner in under 30 minutes using basic ingredients.

Ingredients

Lamb Chops:
- 1 rack lamb chops, sliced and patted dry

Marinade:
- 1 tbsp liquid smoke, 1 tbsp olive oil, 3 cloves garlic (minced)
- 2 tbsp molasses, 1 tbsp paprika, 1 tbsp rosemary (chopped)
- Salt and pepper to taste

Mint Sauce:
- 1 cup fresh mint, ½ cup Greek yogurt, 1 tsp honey
- 1 tsp olive oil, juice of ½ lemon, salt to taste

Additional Toppings:
- 2 peaches (sliced, coated with olive oil and a pinch of salt)
- Balsamic glaze (for drizzling)

Instructions

- Marinate the lamb: combine marinade ingredients. Coat lamb chops and refrigerate for 1 hour.
- Air fry the lamb: preheat air fryer to 400°F. Air fry chops for 10 minutes, flipping halfway.
- Make the mint sauce: blend all mint sauce ingredients until smooth.
- Air fry peaches: coat peach slices with olive oil and salt. Air fry at 375°F for 10 minutes.
- Serve: plate lamb chops with peaches, drizzle with balsamic glaze, and serve with mint sauce on the side.

Scan to watch

Serves 4

Prep time 10 min

Cook time 20 min

Quick Tips:
- No air fryer? Grill the chops—4-5 minutes per side on high.
- Swap mint for cilantro or parsley if desired.
- Serve with roasted veggies or a green salad to complete the meal.

Calories: ~320 | Protein: ~28g | Carbs: ~12g | Fat: ~18g

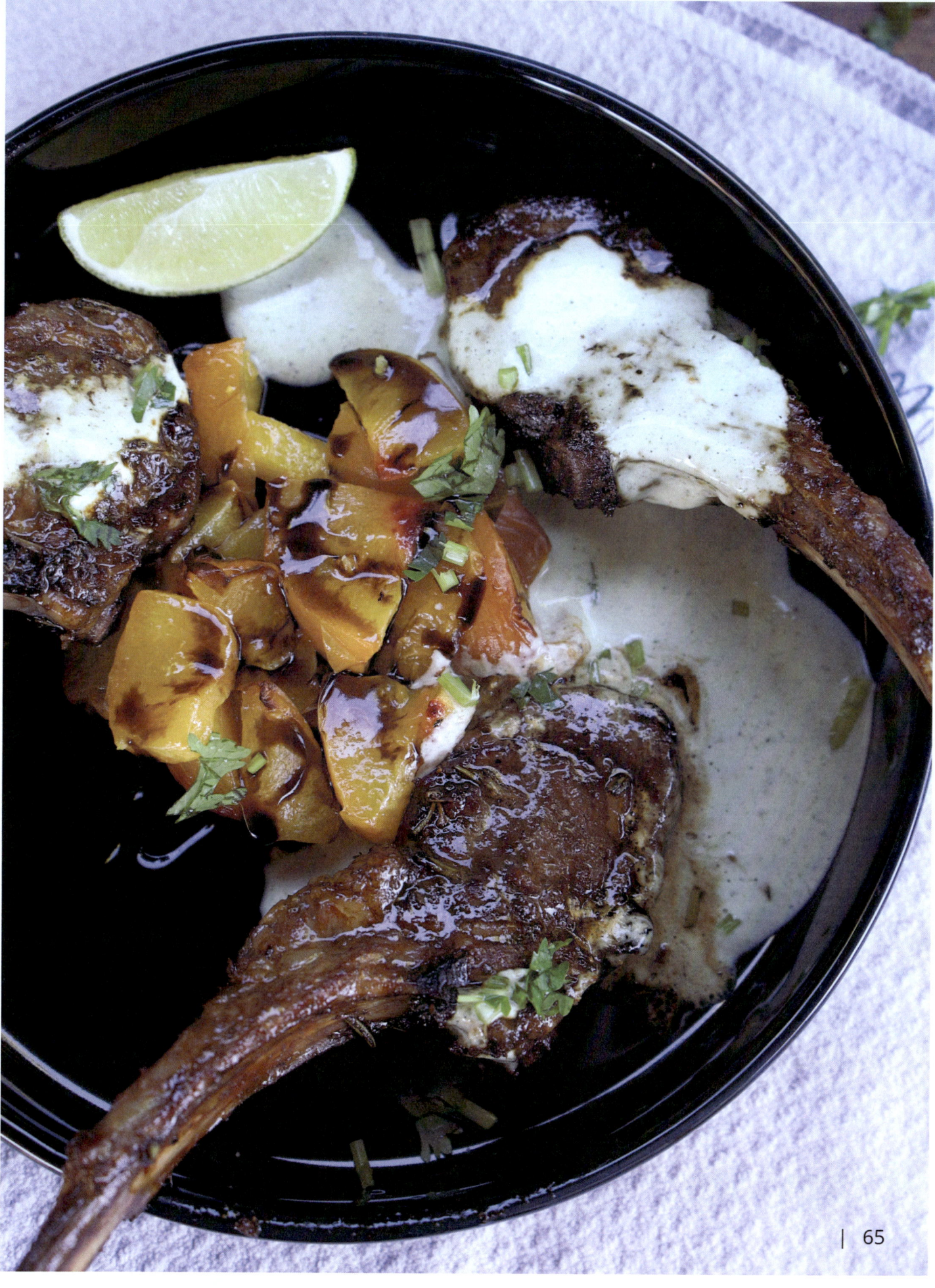

HIGH-PROTEIN WAFFLES WITH ONLY 3 INGREDIENTS

This quick and easy recipe is perfect for a satisfying meal in under 30 minutes, using canned chicken breast as the star ingredient. Recipe makes 8 waffles.

Ingredients

- **2 cups canned chicken breast (or 2 cans of Costco chicken breast)**
- **1 cup shredded cheese (Mexican cheese works great)**
- **2 eggs**

Optional Add-ins:

- ½ cup frozen corn
- 1 jalapeño, chopped
- **Seasonings: salt, pepper, cumin to taste**
- **Oil spray for waffle maker**

Instructions

- Preheat & spray: preheat the waffle maker and lightly spray with oil.
- Mix Ingredients: In a bowl, combine canned chicken, shredded cheese, eggs, and optional add-ins (corn and jalapeño). Season with salt, pepper, and cumin.
- Cook waffles: spoon about 2 tablespoons of the mixture onto the waffle maker and cook for 7 minutes or until crispy and golden.
- Serve: enjoy as-is or turn into a sandwich with your favorite toppings.

Scan to watch

Serves 4

Prep time
5 min

Cook time
7 min

Quick Tips:
- Use other types of cooked chicken breast for this recipe.
- Make the waffles ahead of time and freeze them for a quick meal.
- for the sauce: Chipotle Mayo, Avocado Cream, Cilantro Lime

Per Serving (2 waffles) Protein: ~30g | Calories: ~280 | Carbs: ~6g | Fat: ~16g | Fiber: ~1g .

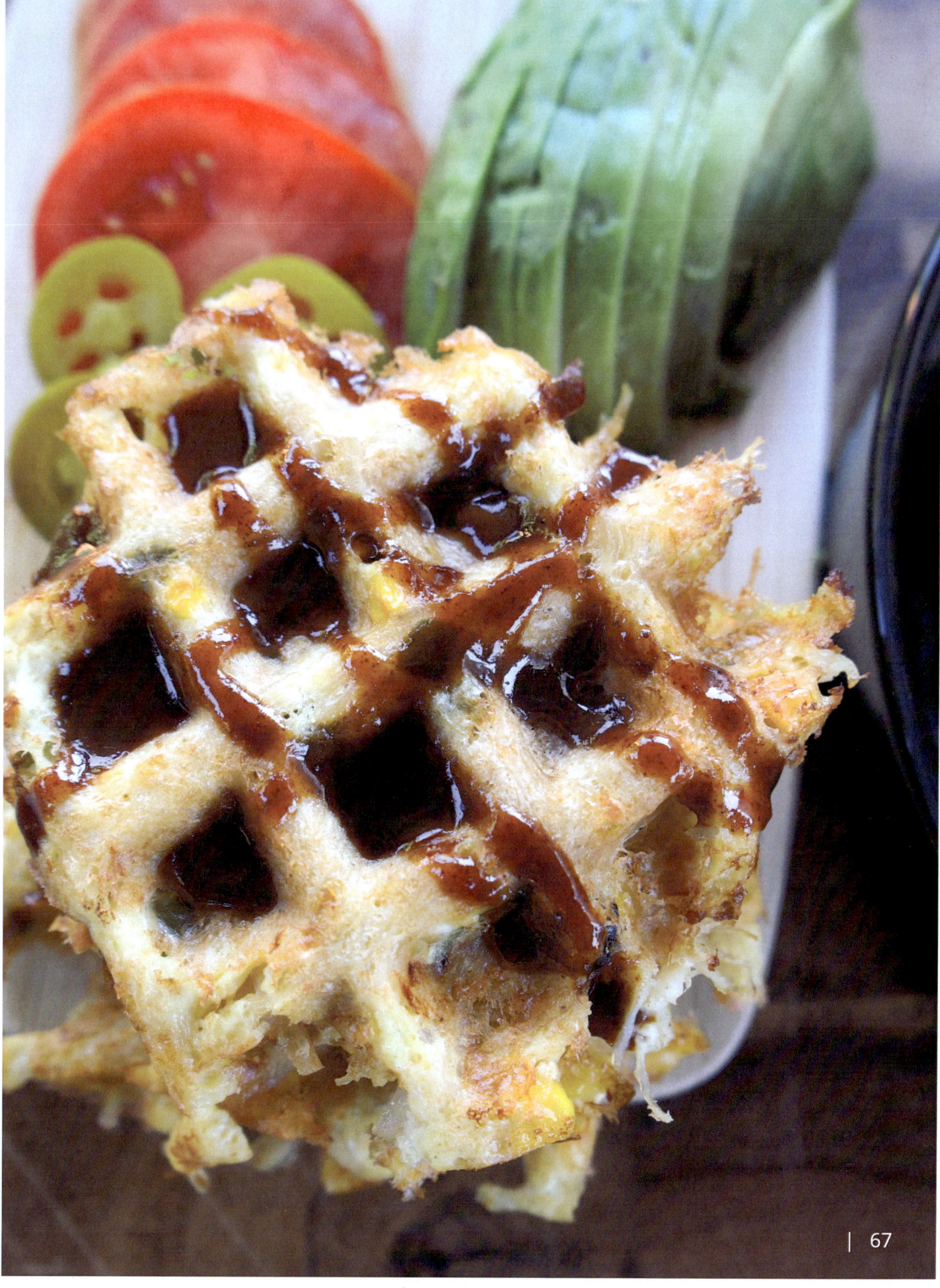

BEST PORK CHOPS IN THE AIR FRYER WITH APPLES AND POTATOES

Air fryer is my best friend—you can make pretty much any dish in it fast, without any extra effort. Just flip halfway, and your dinner is done!

Ingredients

Pork Chops:
- 3 pork chops (6 oz each)

Marinade:
- Salt & pepper to taste
- 1 tsp paprika
- Lemon zest
- 1 tsp garlic powder
- 2 tbsp chopped rosemary
- 1 tbsp Dijon mustard
- 3 tbsp olive oil
- 2 tbsp fruit vinegar

Potatoes:
- 3-4 potatoes
- Salt & pepper, to taste
- 1 tsp garlic powder
- 1 tsp paprika
- 2 tbsp olive oil

Apples:
- 4 apples, sliced
- 2 tbsp honey
- 1 tsp cinnamon
- 1 tbsp lemon juice

Instructions

- Marinate pork chops: mix marinade ingredients, coat pork chops, and refrigerate for 30 minutes.
- Cook pork chops: air fry at 400°F for 12 minutes, flipping halfway, until internal temperature reaches 145°F.
- Prepare potatoes: cut into wedges, season, drizzle with olive oil, and air fry until golden, flipping occasionally.
- Caramelize apples: in a pan, cook apples with honey, cinnamon, and lemon juice until tender and golden.
- Serve: plate pork chops with potatoes and caramelized apples.

Scan to watch

Serves 3

Prep time 10 min

Cook time 20 min

Quick Tips:
- Mix It Up: try pears instead of apples for a twist.
- Let them sit for a few minutes after cooking to lock in juices.
- Add a splash of apple cider to the apples while cooking.

Calories: ~485 | Protein: ~45g | Carbs: ~42g | Fat: ~18g

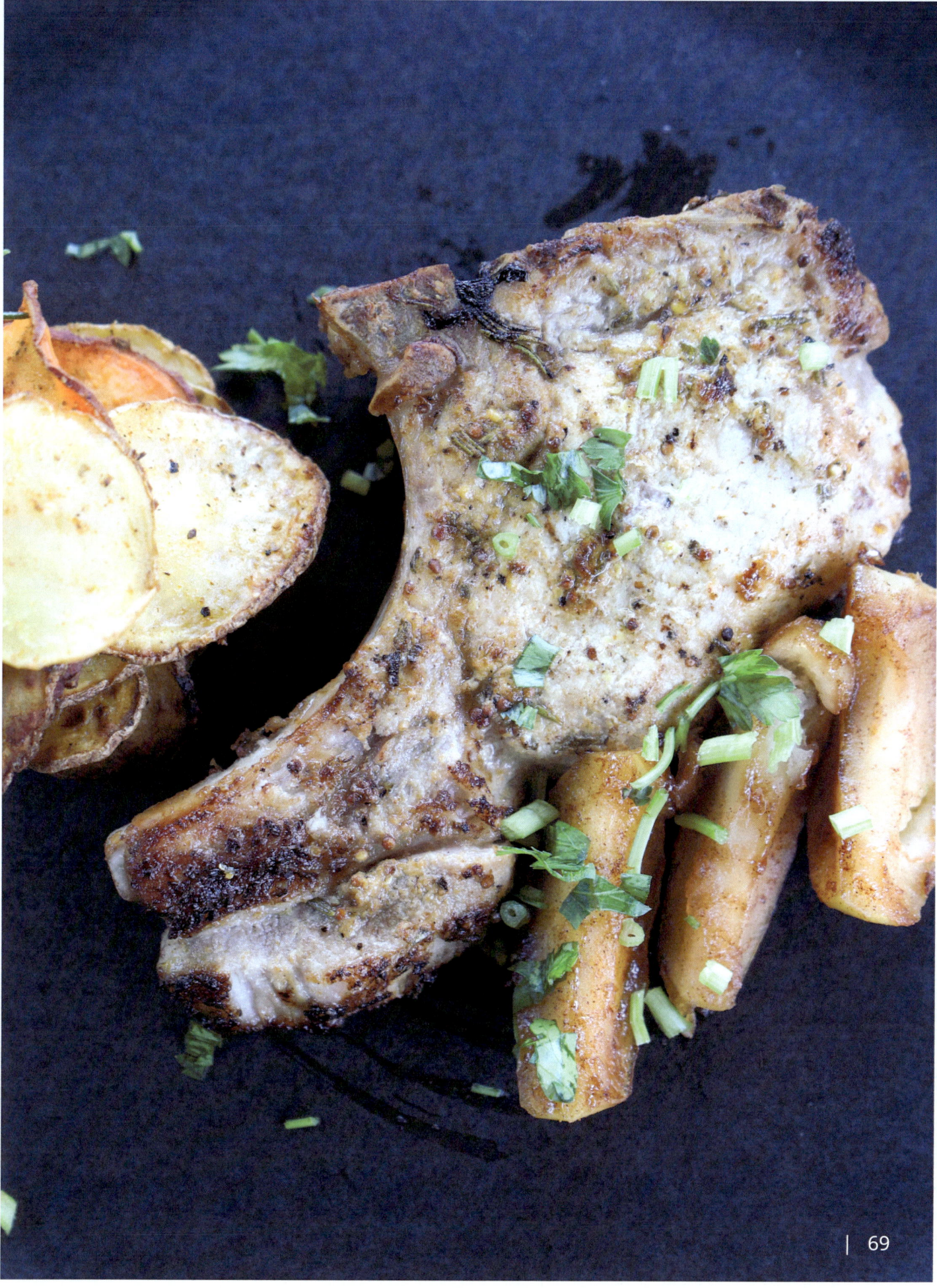

THAI PEANUT SPAGHETTI SQUASH WITH GROUND CHICKEN

A high-protein, low-carb twist on Thai flavors that's hearty, rich, and totally guilt-free. Perfect for when you're craving takeout but want to keep it healthy.

Ingredients

- **1 medium spaghetti squash**
- **1 tbsp olive oil**
- **Salt and pepper to taste**
- **1 lb ground chicken**
- **1 cup shredded carrots**
- **1 cup sliced bell peppers (red or yellow)**
- **3 cups fresh spinach**
- **1/4 cup peanut butter**
- **1 tsp chili paste (adjust for spice)**
- **1 can (13.5 oz) coconut milk**
- **1 tsp fish sauce**
- **1 tbsp coconut aminos**
- **1 tbsp lime juice**
- **1/4 cup chopped cilantro**
- **1/3 cup crushed peanuts (for garnish)**
- **Lime wedges (for serving)**

Instructions

- Cook squash: preheat oven to 400°F or air fryer to 375°F. Roast halved squash for 30-35 minutes (oven) or 25-30 minutes (air fryer). Scrape out strands.
- Brown chicken: cook ground chicken in a skillet over medium heat for 7-10 minutes. Set aside.
- Make sauce: in the same skillet, mix peanut butter, chili paste, coconut milk, fish sauce, coconut aminos, and lime juice. Simmer for 2-3 minutes.
- Cook veggies: add carrots, bell peppers, and spinach to the sauce. Cook until tender (3-5 minutes).
- Combine: toss in chicken and squash. Top with cilantro, peanuts, and lime wedges.

Scan to watch

Serves 4

Prep time 10 min

Cook time 40 min

Quick Tips:
- Microwave squash: to save time, microwave the spaghetti squash for 10-12 minutes instead of roasting. Just poke holes, place it on a plate, and microwave until soft.

Calories: ~450 | Protein: ~30g | Carbs: ~25g | Fat: ~27g

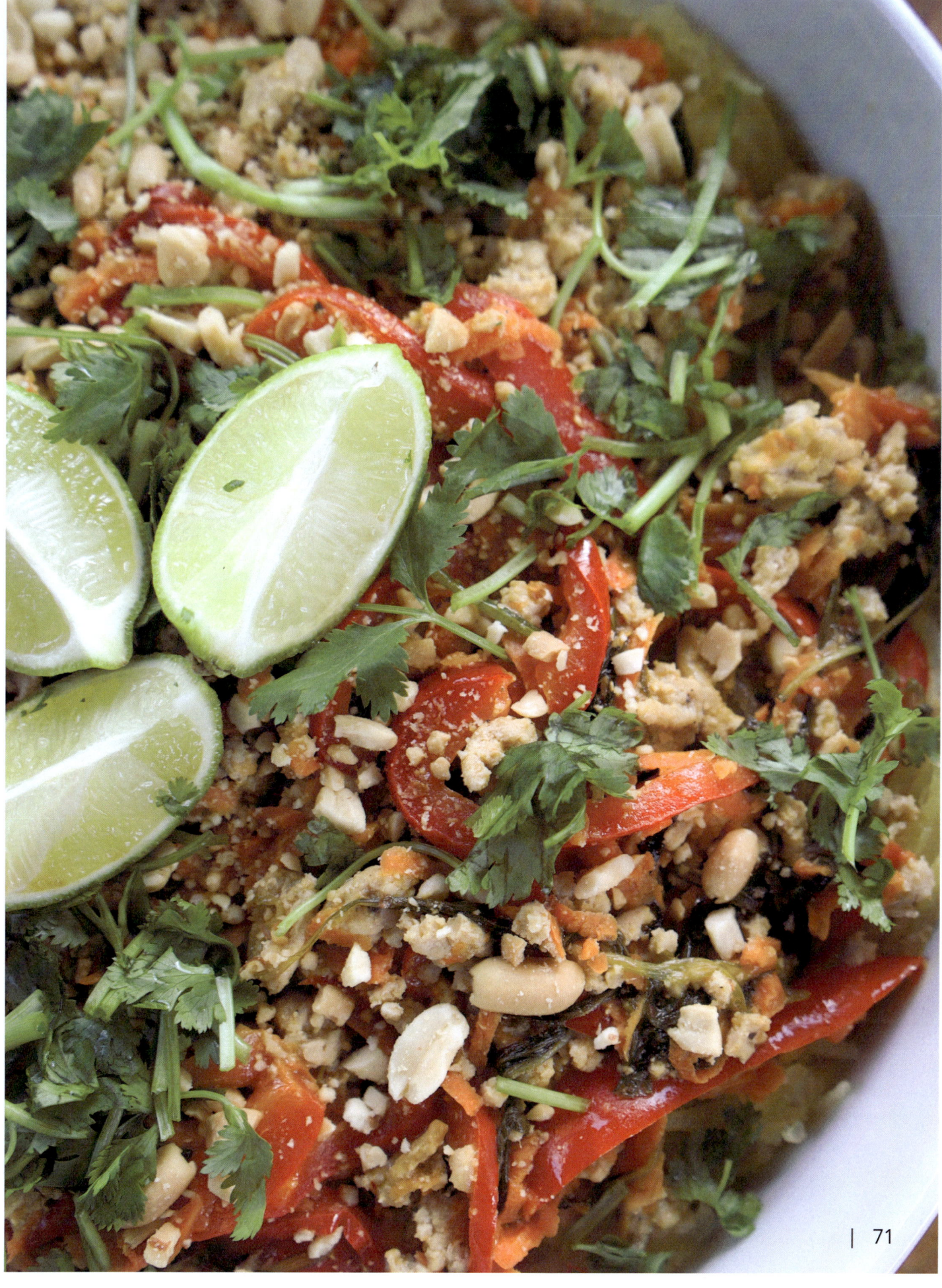

CANNELLINI BEANS PARMESAN BAKE

A high-protein, fall-inspired dish that's warm, hearty, and ready in 30 minutes or less. Perfect for a cozy dinner or lunch, this one-dish wonder can be made vegetarian by skipping the sausage.

Ingredients

- **2 cans cannellini or northern white beans**
- **1 can diced tomatoes**
- **2 tbsp Greek yogurt (optional, for creaminess)**
- **1 onion, chopped**
- **3 cups spinach or kale, chopped**
- **1 cup smoked sausage, chopped**
- **1 cup chicken broth**
- **2 tbsp lemon juice**
- **2 tbsp fruit vinegar**
- **Seasonings: red pepper flakes, garlic powder, salt and pepper to taste**
- **2 cups grated Parmesan cheese**
- **Oil spray**

Instructions

- Preheat oven: preheat to 375°F. Spray a baking dish with oil.
- Layer ingredients: layer the beans, diced tomatoes, onion, spinach or kale, sausage (if using), chicken broth, lemon juice, vinegar, and seasonings in the baking dish. Top with grated Parmesan cheese.
- Bake: cover with foil and bake for 30 minutes. Remove foil halfway through to allow cheese to melt and brown.
- Serve: serve hot with crusty bread for a complete meal.

Scan to watch

Serves 4

Prep time 10 min

Cook time 30 min

Quick Tips:
- Make It vegan: swap the sausage for a plant-based option (like vegan sausage or mushrooms).
- You can prep this dish up to a day in advance, pop it in the oven when you're ready to eat.

400-450 (depending on sausage choice) | Protein: ~25-30g | Carbs: ~30g | Fat: ~18g

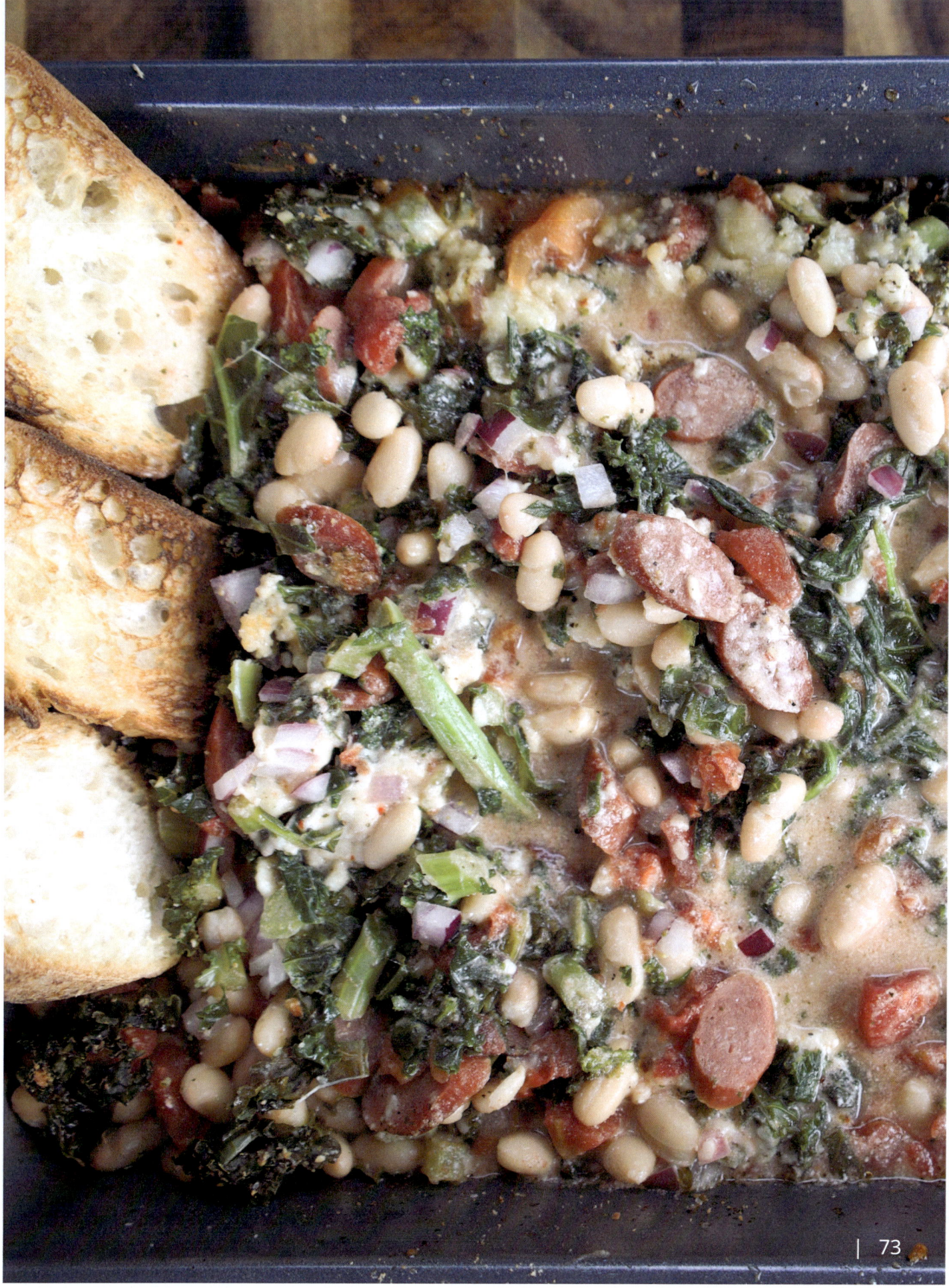

SQUASH AND BEANS GRATIN

Comfort food elevated with high-protein ingredients, perfect for colder fall days. This dish layers tender squash, creamy beans, and gooey cheese for a gratin that's both hearty and satisfying. Add ground meat or sausage for an extra protein boost!

Ingredients

- **2 honey squashes (or any squash of your choice), peeled and thinly sliced**
- **1 onion, thinly sliced**
- **3 garlic cloves, minced**
- **2 tbsp honey mustard**
- **2 cans butter beans, drained**
- **Salt and pepper to taste**
- **½ cup milk**
- **3 tbsp Greek yogurt**
- **1 tsp sage**
- **1 tsp rosemary**
- **Olive oil for sautéing**
- **1 ½ cups grated cheese (Gruyere and Mexican blend)**
- **Optional: 1 lb ground meat or sausage, cooked and seasoned**

Instructions

- Preheat oven to 350°F.
- Prepare squash: slice the squash in half, remove seeds, and cut into slices.
- Sauté onions and garlic: heat olive oil in a skillet over medium heat. Sauté onions for 3 minutes, then add garlic and cook for 1 more minute.
- Make the bean mixture: stir in honey mustard, butter beans, milk, Greek yogurt, and seasonings. Simmer for 5 minutes on medium-low heat.
- Layer in a baking dish: start with a layer of squash, followed by beans and cheese. If using meat, add it after the beans. Repeat the layers.
- Bake: cover with foil and bake for 40 minutes. Remove foil and bake for another 5 minutes

Scan to watch

Serves 6

Prep time 15 min

Cook time 55 min

Quick Tips:
- Add a scoop of cottage cheese or ricotta between the layers for extra protein and creaminess.
- You can slice the squash and prepare the bean mixture the night before.

Without meat: 315-350 | Protein: ~16g | Carbs: ~35g | Fat: ~14g
With meat: 420-450 | Protein: ~28g | Carbs: ~35g | Fat: ~22g

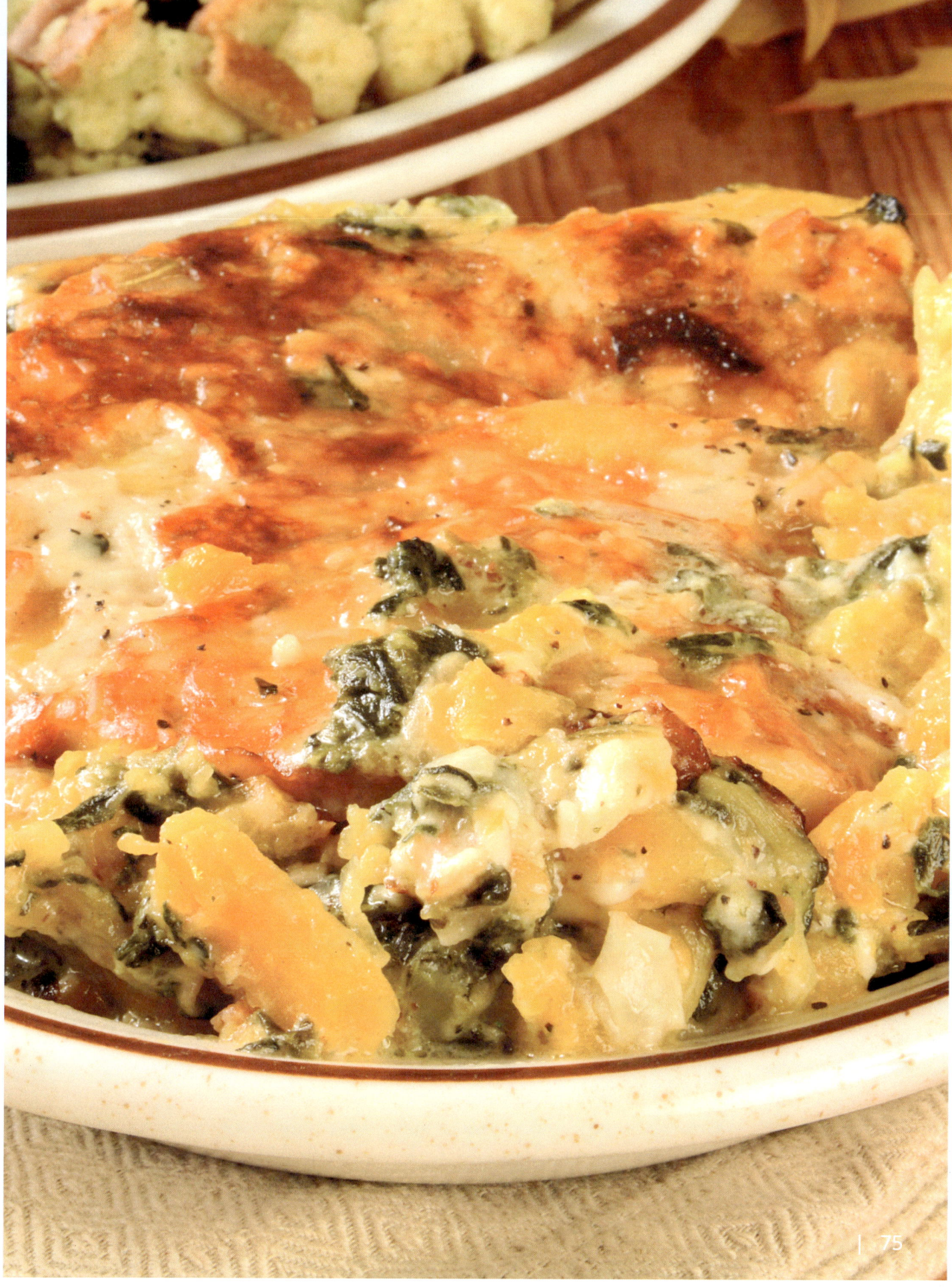

HIGH-PROTEIN LAMB VINDALOO

This high-protein Lamb Vindaloo is a family favorite—my wife's top pick whenever we order at restaurants. Now, I've brought this flavorful, spicy dish home, and it's ready in under 40 minutes using the Instant Pot. With its bold flavors, this dish is a tasty tribute to the classic Indian Vindaloo, originally brought to India by Portuguese colonists.

Ingredients

- **1 lb lamb shoulder (cubed)**
- **1 large onion (chopped)**
- **6 potatoes (sliced)**
- **2–3 tsp chili powder**
- **3 tsp ginger garlic paste**
- **2 tsp toasted cumin seeds (ground)**
- **1 tsp black pepper**
- **2 tsp toasted cloves (ground)**
- **4 cinnamon sticks**
- **4 bay leaves**
- **1 tsp sumac**
- **3 tbsp olive oil**
- **Juice of 1 lime**
- **3 tsp tomato paste**
- **1 cup water**
- **Salt to taste**
- **Parsley (for garnish)**

Instructions

- Marinate: blend cumin, cloves, chili powder, ginger garlic paste, sumac, olive oil, lime juice, tomato paste, and black pepper into a smooth paste. Coat lamb cubes in the marinade and refrigerate for 3–4 hours.
- Cook: sauté onions in olive oil in the Instant Pot until soft. Add marinated lamb, cinnamon sticks, and bay leaves. Sauté for 2-3 minutes. Add sliced potatoes and water. Seal the lid and cook on high pressure for 40 minutes. Let pressure release naturally.
- Serve: garnish with parsley and serve hot, ideally with rice.

Scan to watch

Serves 4

Prep time
10 min

Cook time
1 h 15 min

Quick Tips:
- For even richer flavor, try using bone-in lamb shoulder.
- To cook on the stove, simmer everything in a large pot over medium heat for 1.5–2 hours, until lamb is tender.

Calories: 650 | Protein: 35g | Carbs: 50g | Fat: 35g

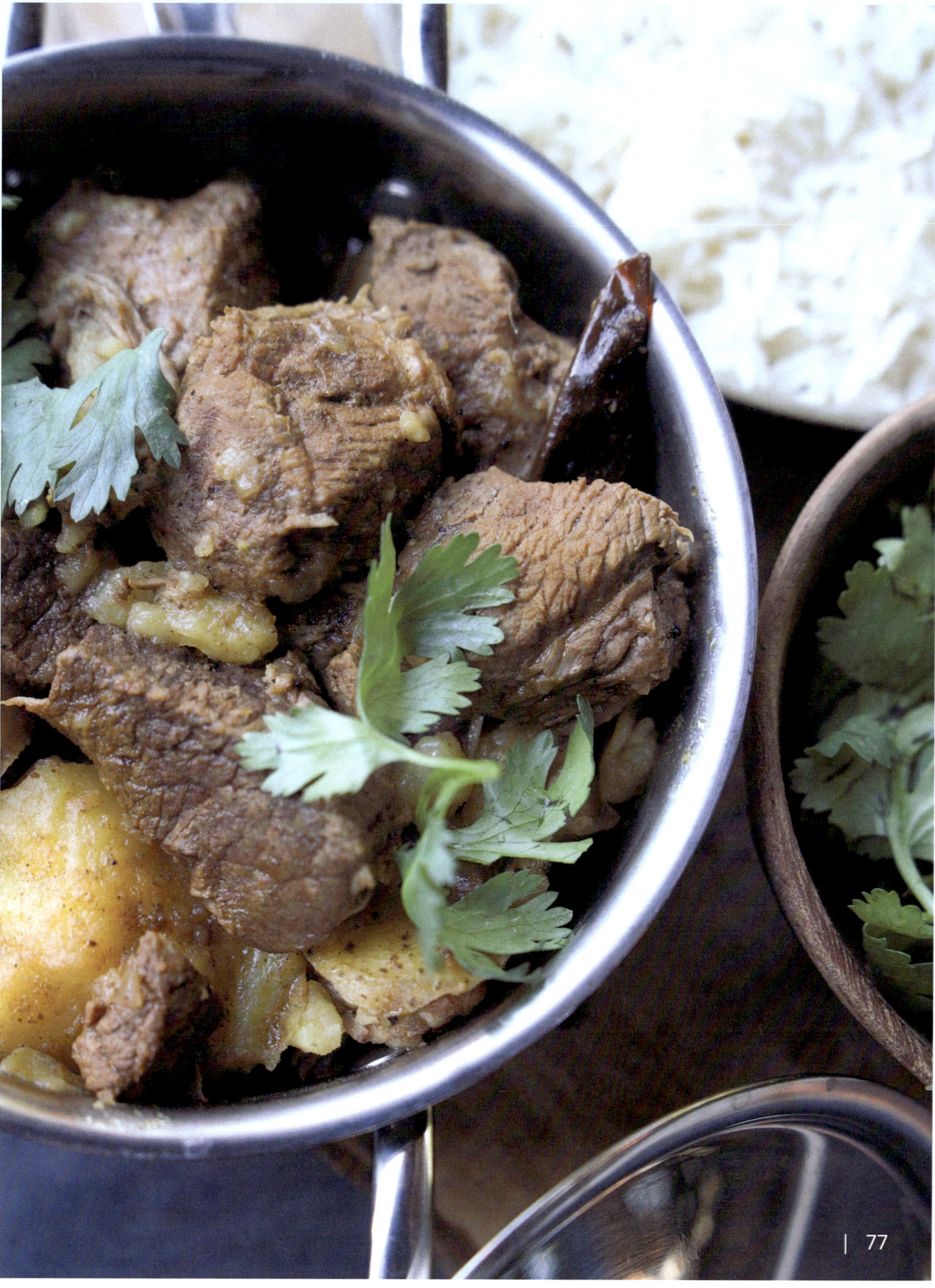

ROASTED CAULIFLOWER WITH TAHINI AND SALSA

Who says low-carb can't be flavorful? This Whole Roasted Cauliflower gets a tangy twist with creamy tahini and fresh salsa. It's like the cauliflower came to the party with a whole new vibe—and it's ready in 30 minutes. Perfect for those days when you want to impress without breaking a sweat.

Ingredients

- **1 whole cauliflower head**
- **1 tbsp lemon juice**
- **Salt & pepper to taste**
- **3 tbsp fruit vinegar (divided) – I'm using my favorite Laconiko products**
- **3 tbsp extra virgin olive oil**
- **3 tbsp tahini paste**
- **3 garlic cloves, minced**
- **3 tsp lemon juice (for tahini sauce)**
- **½ cup parsley, chopped (divided)**
- **2 cups tomatoes, chopped**
- **¼ cup jalapeños, chopped**
- **½ cup red onion, chopped**
- **2 tbsp lime juice**
- **1 cup Greek yogurt (for serving)**

Instructions

- Steam cauliflower in the Instant Pot with 1 cup water on manual mode for 0 minutes. Quick release.
- Roast: preheat oven to 400°F. Drizzle cauliflower with lemon juice, 2 tbsp olive oil, 2 tbsp vinegar, salt, and pepper. Roast for 15-20 minutes until golden.
- Tahini sauce: mix tahini, 3 tsp lemon juice, garlic, and 1 tbsp olive oil. Add water to achieve a smooth consistency. Stir in ¼ cup parsley.
- Salsa: combine tomatoes, jalapeños, onion, lime juice, 1 tbsp vinegar, and remaining parsley.
- Serve: spread Greek yogurt on a plate, top with cauliflower, drizzle with tahini, and finish with salsa.

Scan to watch

Serves 4

Prep time
10 min

Cook time
20 min

Quick Tips:
- Steam cauliflower for a tender inside and crispy exterior
- Broil the cauliflower for 2-3 minutes at the end to get a crispy, caramelized top.

Calories: 250 | Protein: 12g | Carbs: 15g | Fat: 18g

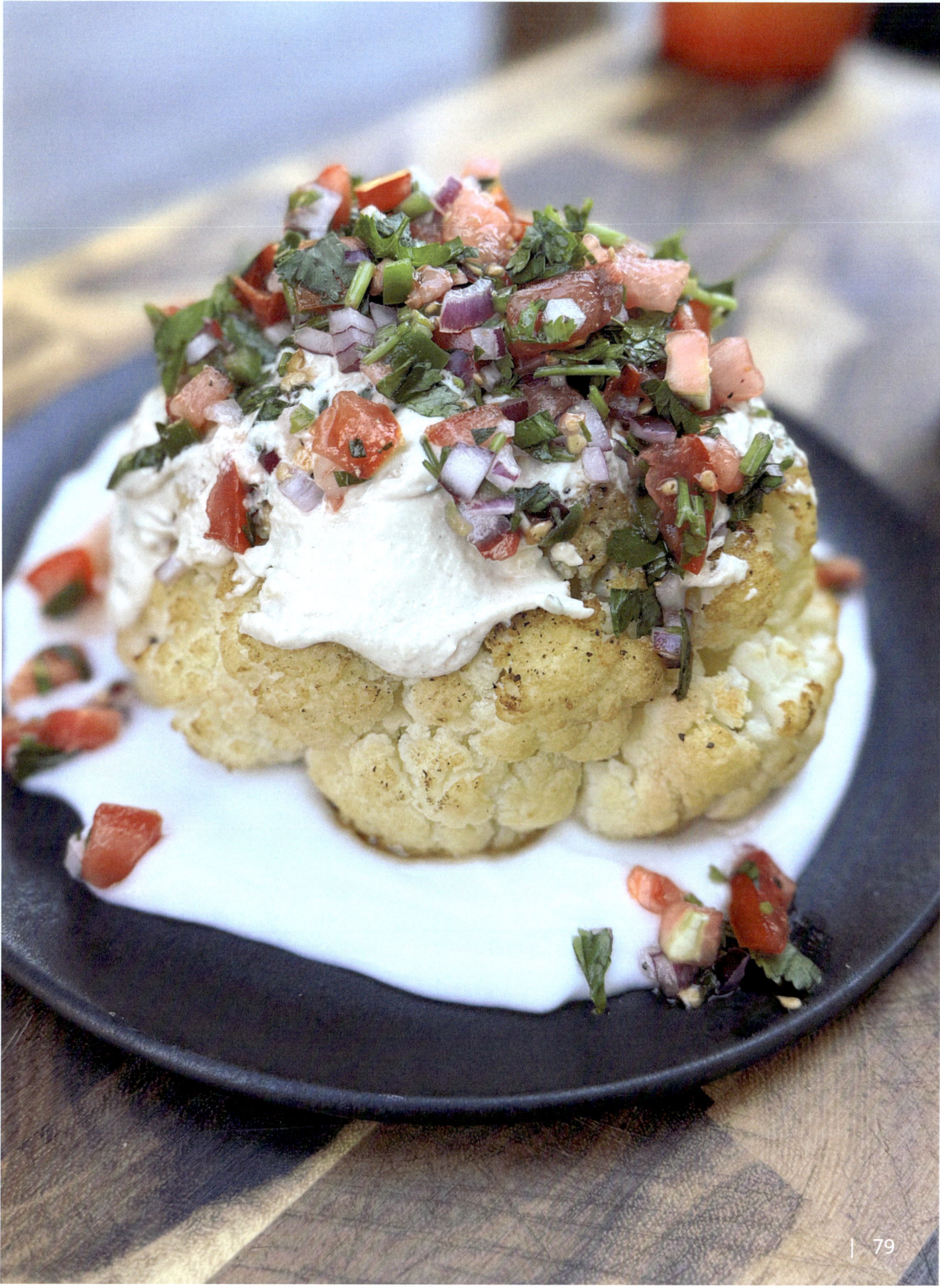

ZUCCHINI PACKETS

This dish is fancy enough for guests yet simple enough for a quick meal. Whether you assemble elegant zucchini packets or throw everything into a skillet, it's packed with flavor and comfort.

Ingredients

- **2 zucchinis (sliced into thin strips with a potato peeler)**
- **1 onion, chopped**
- **6 garlic cloves, minced (divided)**
- **3 cups mushrooms, chopped**
- **1 lb ground turkey**
- **3 cups spinach**
- **½ cup ricotta cheese**
- **1 can (14 oz) San Marzano tomatoes**
- **1 tbsp oil**
- **Fresh basil leaves**
- **Seasoning: cumin, sumac, hot paprika, salt, pepper, chili powder (to taste)**
- **Toppings: grated Parmesan, fresh basil**

Instructions

- Cook the filling: heat oil in a skillet. Sauté onions until soft, then add half the garlic, mushrooms, turkey, and spinach and seasoning, cook until browned.
- Assemble packets: lay zucchini strips in a grid (3-4 vertical, 3-4 horizontal). Add a spoonful of meat filling, a teaspoon of ricotta, and fold into a packet. Makes ~15 packets.
- Make the sauce: in the same skillet, heat oil, sauté remaining garlic, then add tomatoes, basil, salt, and chili powder. Simmer until slightly thickened.
- Cook the packets: nestle packets into the sauce, cover, and simmer for 10 minutes.
- Serve: plate 3 packets per serving, topped with Parmesan and fresh basil.

Scan to watch

Serves 5

Prep time
15 min

Cook time
15 min

Quick Tips:
- Skip the packets: for a faster meal, toss everything on the skillet or Instant Pot and cook on high pressure for 3 minutes.

Calories: 290 | Protein: 28g | Carbs: 16g | Fat: 12g

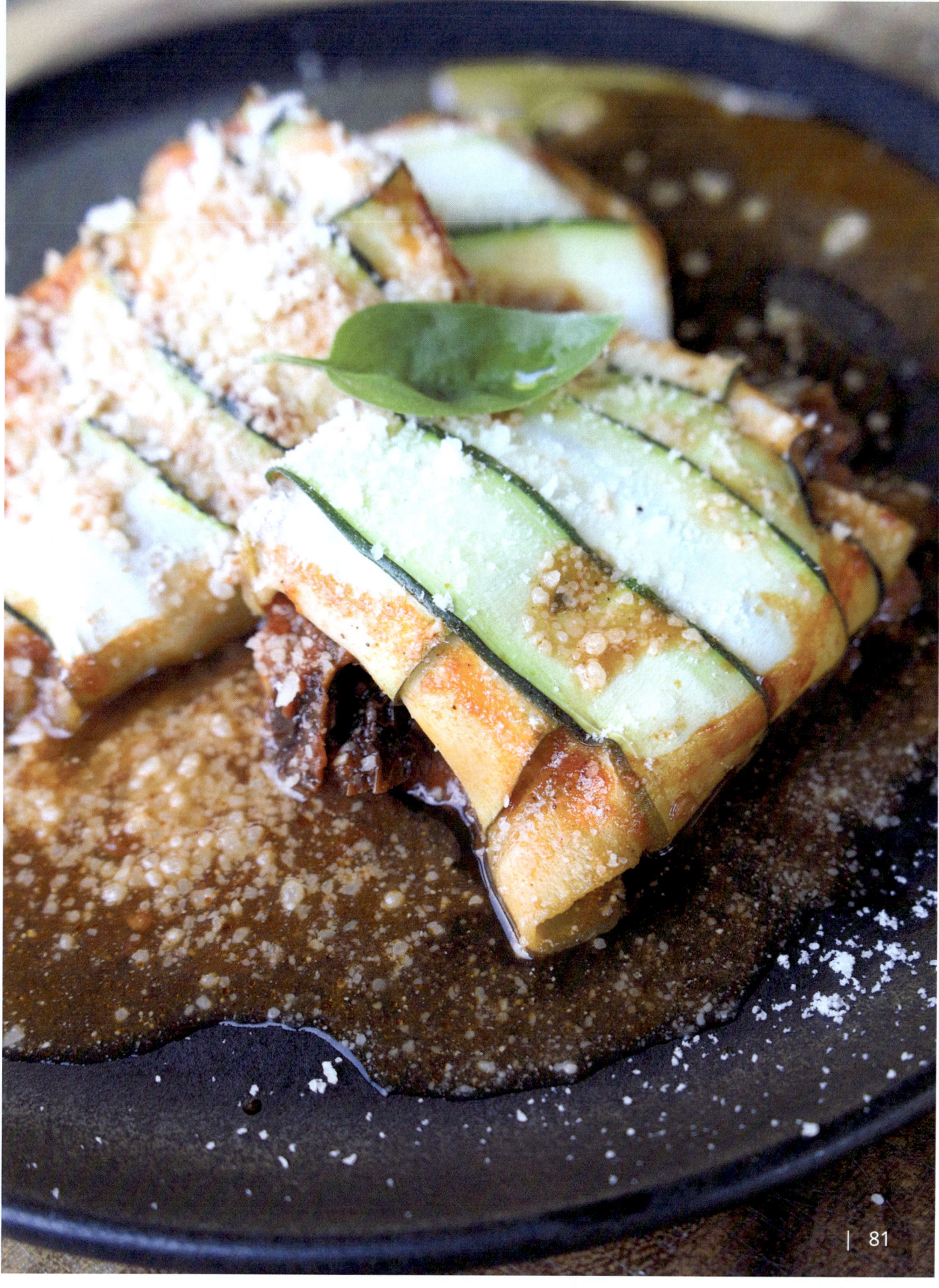

GOCHUJANG CHICKEN WINGS

These wings are the ultimate balance of heat, sweetness, and umami, with an air-fried crisp that keeps them light yet flavorful. Toss them in sauce after cooking for that perfect texture—trust me, it makes all the difference!

Ingredients

- **2 lb chicken wings**
- **2½ tbsp gochujang (Korean chili paste)**
- **2 tsp soy sauce**
- **1 tbsp mayonnaise**
- **1 tbsp toasted sesame oil**
- **2 tsp ginger-garlic paste**
- **2½ tbsp honey**
- **Salt and pepper, to taste**
- **Oil spray (for air frying)**
- **1 tsp sesame seeds, for garnish**
- **¼ cup chopped scallions, for garnish**

Instructions

- Season & air fry: preheat air fryer to 360°F. Season wings with salt and pepper, lightly spray the air fryer basket with oil, and cook for 20-25 min, flipping halfway through.
- Make the sauce: while wings cook, whisk together gochujang, soy sauce, mayonnaise, sesame oil, ginger & garlic paste, and honey.
- Toss in sauce: when wings reach 160°F, toss them in half the sauce (this keeps them crispy!).
- Final crisp: return to the air fryer for 5 min at 400°F until the sauce caramelizes.
- Serve & garnish: top with sesame seeds and scallions. Serve with remaining sauce for dipping.

Scan to watch

Serves 4

Prep time
5 min

Cook time
25 min

Quick Tips:
- For extra-crispy wings, pat them dry before air frying, and always toss in sauce after cooking—never before!

Calories: 320 | Protein: 32g | Carbs: 14g | Fat: 16g

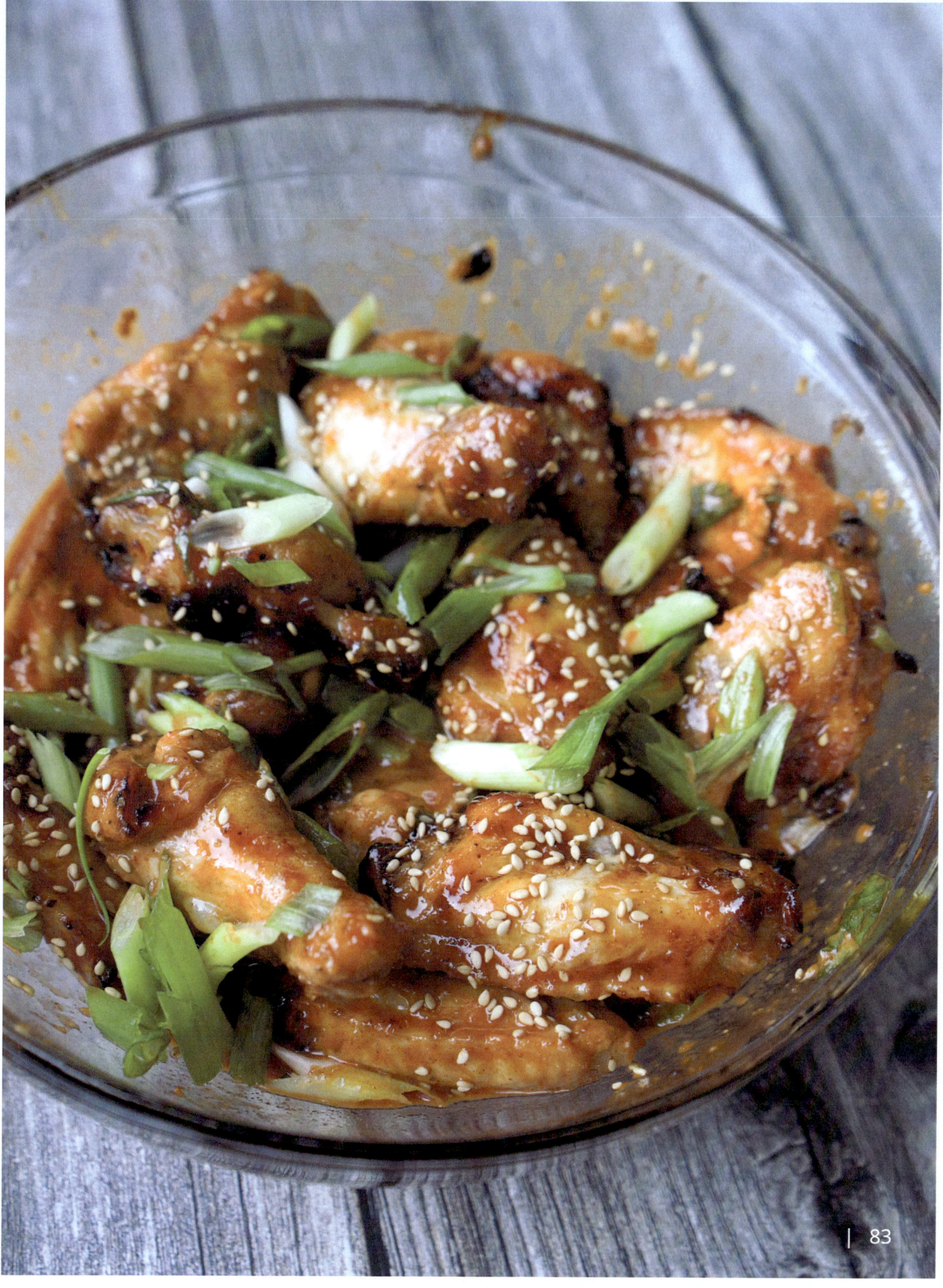

TURKEY SLIDERS WITH CRANBERRY SAUCE

These turkey sliders are your new go-to for parties, potlucks, or just an easy weeknight meal. The mix of melty cheese, crispy bacon, and tangy cranberry sauce makes them unreal. Bonus: they're ready in just 15 minutes!

Ingredients

- **6 Hawaiian slider buns**
- **12 oz sliced turkey**
- **½ cup cranberry sauce (homemade or store-bought)**
- **1 cup shredded cheese (Gruyère and Mexican blend recommended)**
- **3 tbsp honey mustard sauce (Trader Joe's Magnifisauce or your favorite)**
- **6 fried bacon strips**
- **1 tsp sesame seeds**
- **Oil spray for toasting**

Instructions

- Prep & assemble: preheat oven to 350°F. Slice buns in half and arrange on a baking sheet.
- Layer: spread cranberry sauce on the bottom half. Add turkey slices, shredded cheese, honey mustard sauce, and crispy bacon.
- Toast & bake: place the bun tops back on, spray lightly with oil, and sprinkle with sesame seeds. Cover with foil and bake for 10 min, removing foil for the last 2 min to toast.
- Serve warm & devour: best enjoyed fresh, but leftovers reheat well in the oven or air fryer.

Scan to watch

Serves 6

Prep time
5 min

Cook time
10 min

Quick Tips:
- Assemble sliders ahead of time and bake just before serving.
- Want a crispier finish? Skip the foil and bake uncovered for the full 10 minutes!

1 Slider: Calories: 219 | Protein: 21g | Carbs: 24g | Fat: 6g

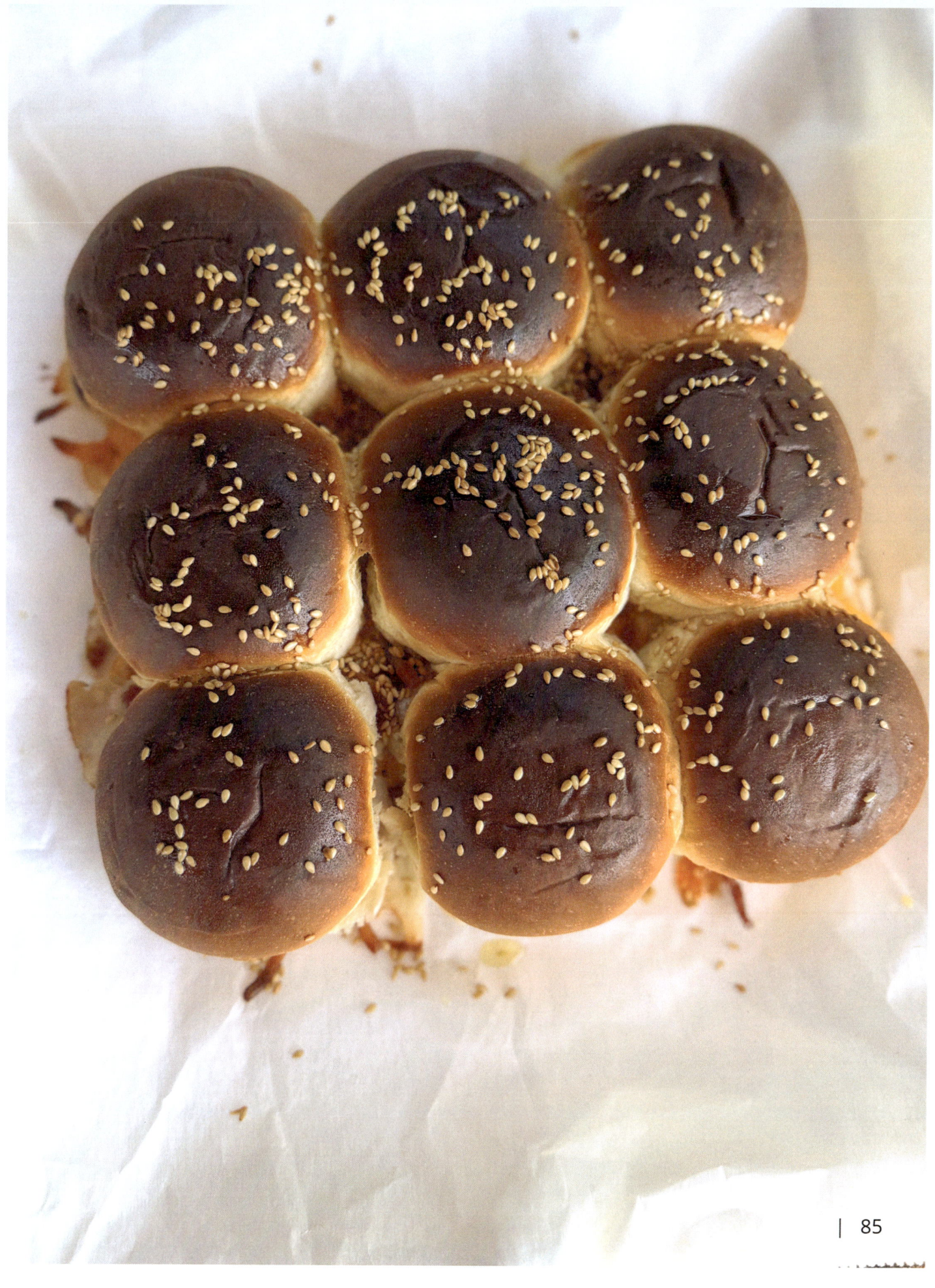

LOW-CARB EGGPLANT LASAGNA

Love lasagna but not the carbs? This version swaps noodles for roasted eggplant, keeping it high in protein and rich in flavor. It's the perfect post-workout meal or cozy comfort food without the guilt.

Ingredients

- **1-2 large eggplants, sliced ¼ inch thick**
- **1 lb ground beef**
- **1 onion, chopped**
- **3 cloves garlic, minced**
- **1 can (14 oz) San Marzano tomatoes**
- **1 tsp Italian seasoning**
- **1 tsp cumin**
- **Salt & pepper to taste**
- **1 tbsp olive oil**
- **1 cup ricotta cheese**
- **1 cup shredded Gruyère cheese**
- **½ cup Parmesan cheese**
- **1 cup cherry tomatoes, halved**
- **Fresh basil for garnish**

Instructions

- Prep eggplant: preheat oven to 425°F. Arrange eggplant slices on a baking sheet, drizzle with olive oil, season with salt & pepper, and roast for 15-20 minutes. Short on time? Microwave eggplant slices for 3-4 minutes to soften before roasting.
- Cook meat sauce: heat oil in a pan, sauté onion and garlic until fragrant. Add ground beef, cook until browned. Stir in San Marzano tomatoes, Italian seasoning, cumin, salt & pepper. Simmer for 5 minutes.
- Assemble lasagna: In a greased baking dish, layer roasted eggplant, meat sauce, ricotta, and basil. Repeat. Top with Gruyère, Parmesan, and cherry tomatoes.
- Bake & serve: bake at 375°F for 15 minutes or until cheese is golden.

Scan to watch

Serves 5

Prep time 10 min

Cook time 30 min

Quick Tips:
- Salt eggplant slices and let them sit for 10 minutes to draw out excess water before roasting.
- Swap Gruyère for mozzarella or add cottage cheese for extra protein.

Calories: 310 | Protein: 27g | Carbs: 14g | Fat: 18g

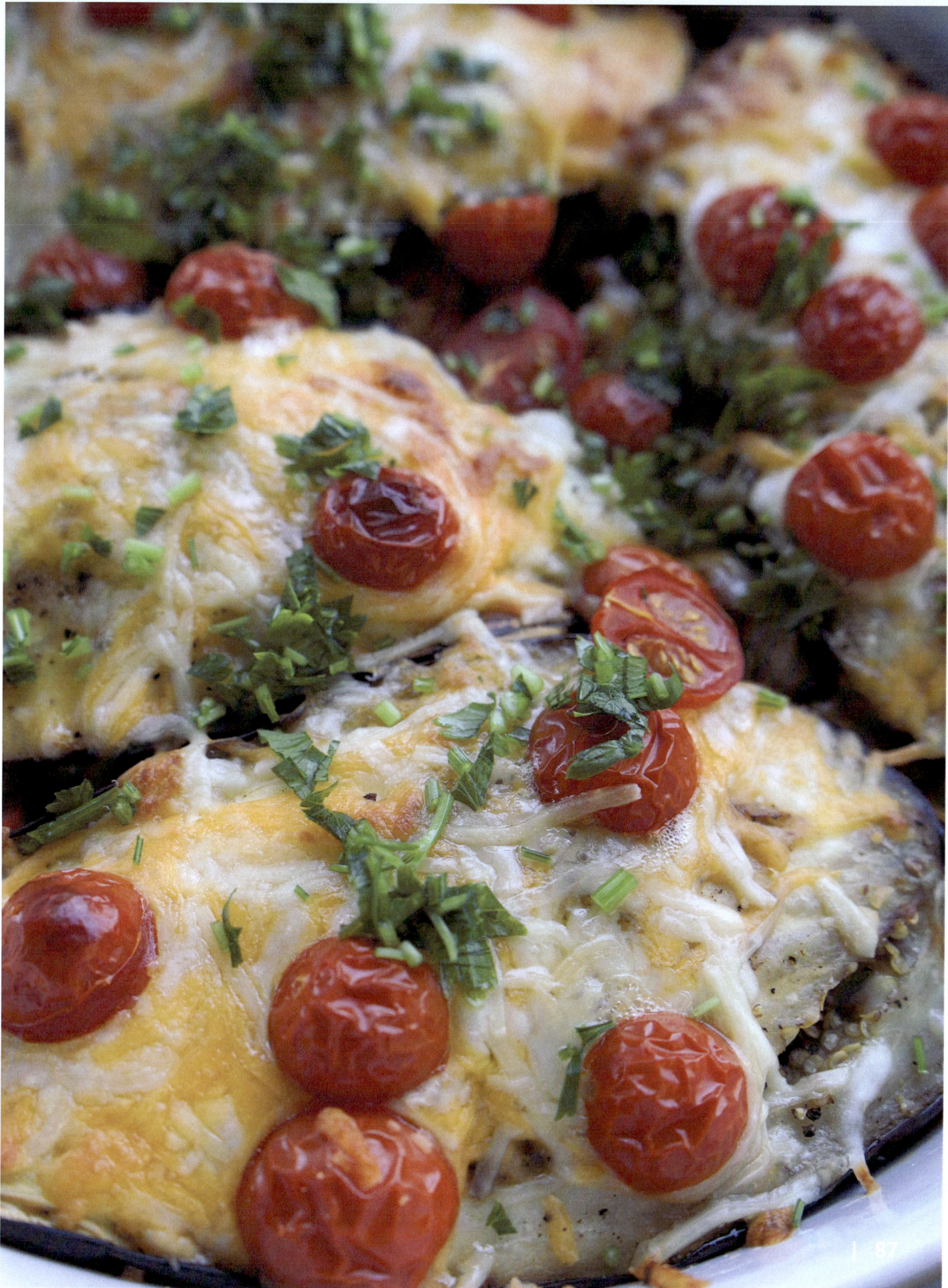

MEAT-STUFFED POTATOES

The first time I made this for a family dinner, the compliments were flying in like I was a Michelin-star chef. Use both yellow and sweet potatoes, or go rogue with whatever you have lying around. Either way, prepare for some serious comfort food vibes.

Ingredients

- **9 yellow potatoes, peeled, parboiled, and halved**
- **5 sweet potatoes, peeled, parboiled, and halved**
- **1 lb ground beef**
- **1 cup parsley, chopped**
- **1 onion, chopped**
- **1 tsp chili powder**
- **1 tsp cumin**
- **1 tsp garlic powder**
- **1 tsp salt**
- **½ tsp pepper**
- **⅓ cup water**
- **25 oz marinara sauce**
- **1 ½ cups cherry tomatoes**
- **1 ½ cups mushrooms**
- **2 cups shredded Mexican or Gruyère cheese**
- **Olive oil, for drizzling**

Instructions

- Parboil the potatoes (yellow and sweet) for about 5 minutes in the Instant Pot, then slice them in half.
- In a bowl, mix ground beef, parsley, onion, seasonings, and water.
- Drizzle half of the marinara sauce in a large baking dish. Take two potato halves and sandwich them around a scoop of the meat mixture. Repeat with all potatoes.
- Pour the remaining marinara sauce over the stuffed potatoes. Scatter cherry tomatoes and mushrooms on top. Drizzle with olive oil.
- Cover with foil and bake at 400°F for 50 minutes. At the 40-minute mark, remove foil, sprinkle cheese on top, and bake uncovered until melty and golden.

Scan to watch

Serves 6

Prep time
15 min

Cook time
50 min

Quick Tips:
- Parboil potatoes in your Instant Pot for 5 minutes on high pressure with a quick release—cuts cooking time in half!
- Swap some potatoes for roasted eggplant or zucchini for a lower-carb twist with the same hearty vibes.

3 Potatoes: Calories: 500 | Protein: 28g | Carbs: 45g | Fat: 20g

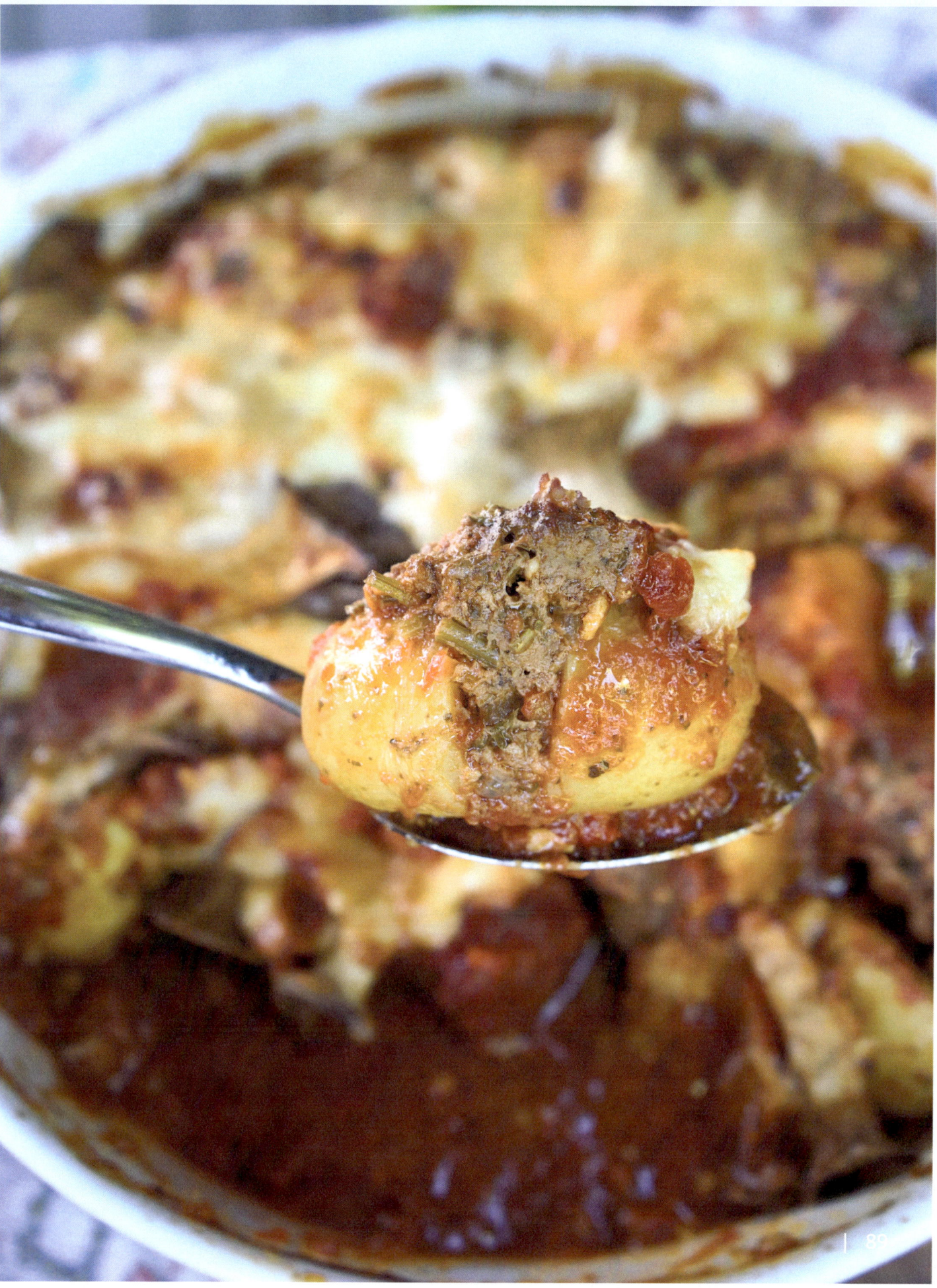

STUFFED SPAGHETTI SQUASH

So, you bought spaghetti squash thinking you'd make some "healthy pasta" dish, but it's been sitting on your counter like a forgotten vegetable. This recipe is here to save your squash from being a countertop decoration.

Ingredients

- **1 medium spaghetti squash (poke holes with a knife and microwave for 10 minutes to make slicing easier)**
- **1 cup cannellini beans, drained and rinsed**
- **1 cup feta cheese**
- **1 cup cherry tomatoes, halved**
- **½ cup fresh parsley, chopped**
- **½ cup pine nuts**
- **Extra virgin olive oil**
- **Fruit vinegar**
- **Salt and pepper to taste**

Instructions

- Microwave & prep: poke holes in the spaghetti squash with a knife and microwave for 10 minutes on high. (This step is a life-saver, trust me.)
- Cut & scoop: slice the spaghetti squash in half lengthwise and scoop out the seeds.
- Stuff it: fill the squash halves with beans, feta, tomatoes, parsley, and pine nuts.
- Drizzle & season: drizzle with olive oil and vinegar, then season with salt and pepper.
- Bake time: bake at 400°F for 20 minutes.

Scan to watch

Serves 4

Prep time
10 min

Cook time
30 min

Quick Tips:
- Microwaving the squash first softens it and reducing overall cooking time.
- Toast the pine nuts beforehand for extra depth of flavor.

Calories: 400 | Protein: 17g | Carbs: 45g | Fat: 20g

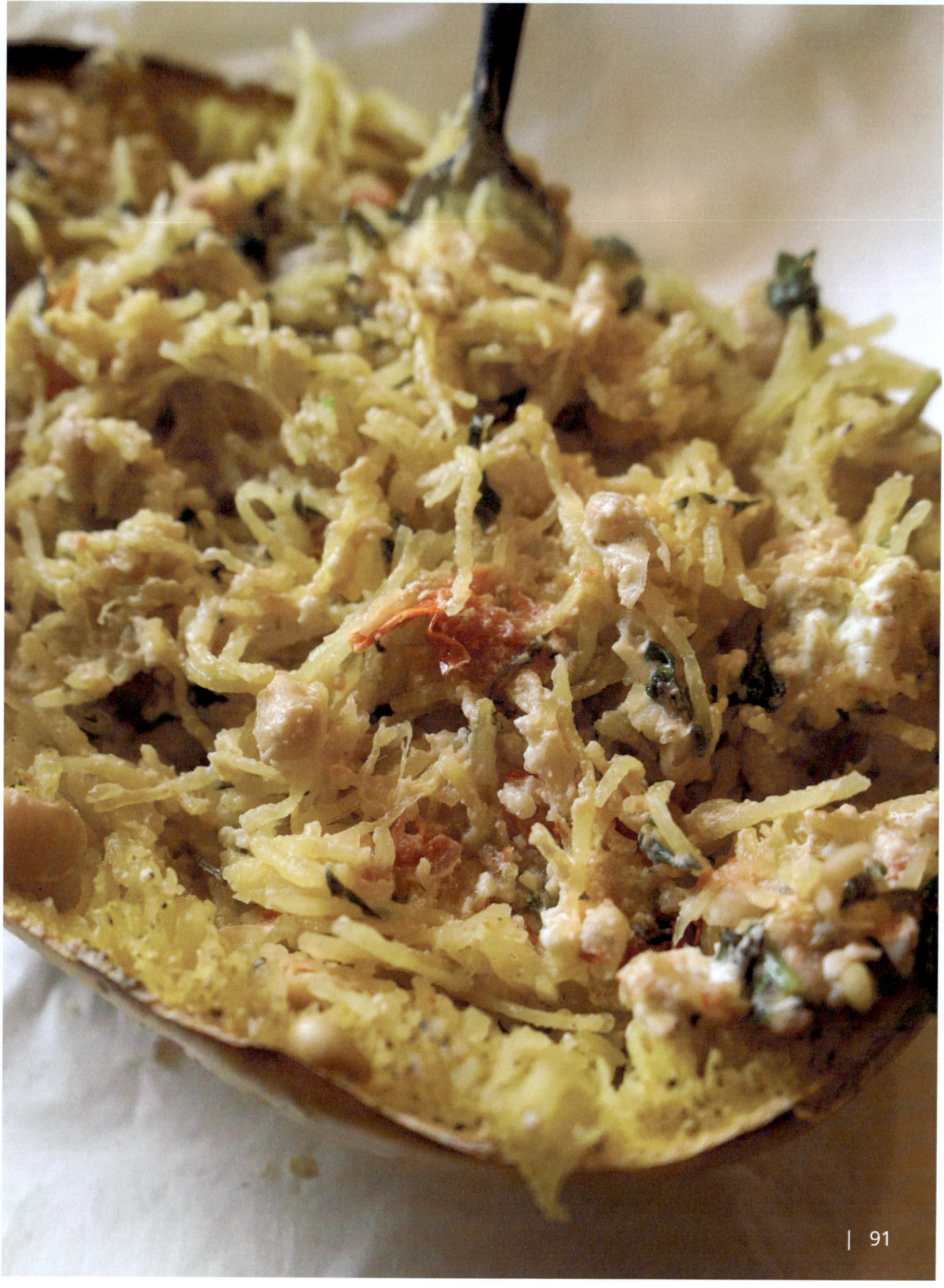

TIKKA MASALA CASSEROLE

This is a fun, no-fuss recipe for those days when you want something delicious without a ton of effort. Spaghetti squash on its own doesn't have much taste, but mix it with a rich, creamy tikka masala sauce, and you'll be reaching for this dish every night.

Ingredients

- **1 medium spaghetti squash (poke holes with a knife and microwave for 10-15 minutes for easy slicing)**
- **Salt & pepper, to taste**
- **Extra virgin olive oil**
- **1.5 lb boneless chicken thighs, cut into smaller pieces**
- **25 oz Tikka Masala sauce (Costco's version is a winner!)**
- **2 tbsp mango chutney**
- **2 bell peppers, chopped**
- **1 large carrot, chopped**
- **1 large onion, thinly sliced**
- **Fresh parsley for garnish**

Instructions

- Prep the squash: microwave the spaghetti squash for 10-15 minutes, slice in half, scoop out seeds, drizzle with oil, season, and roast at 400°F for 15 minutes.
- Cook the chicken: cut chicken, season, coat with Tikka Masala sauce.
- Layer & bake: in a casserole dish, layer spaghetti squash strands, chicken, and veggies. Repeat, season top layer, cover with foil, and bake at 375°F for 25-30 minutes until chicken reaches 165°F.

Scan to watch

Serves 6

Prep time 15 min

Cook time 45 min

Quick Tips:
- Stir a spoonful of Greek yogurt or coconut cream into the Tikka Masala sauce for added creaminess.

Calories: 380 | Protein: 27g | Carbs: 22g | Fat: 15g

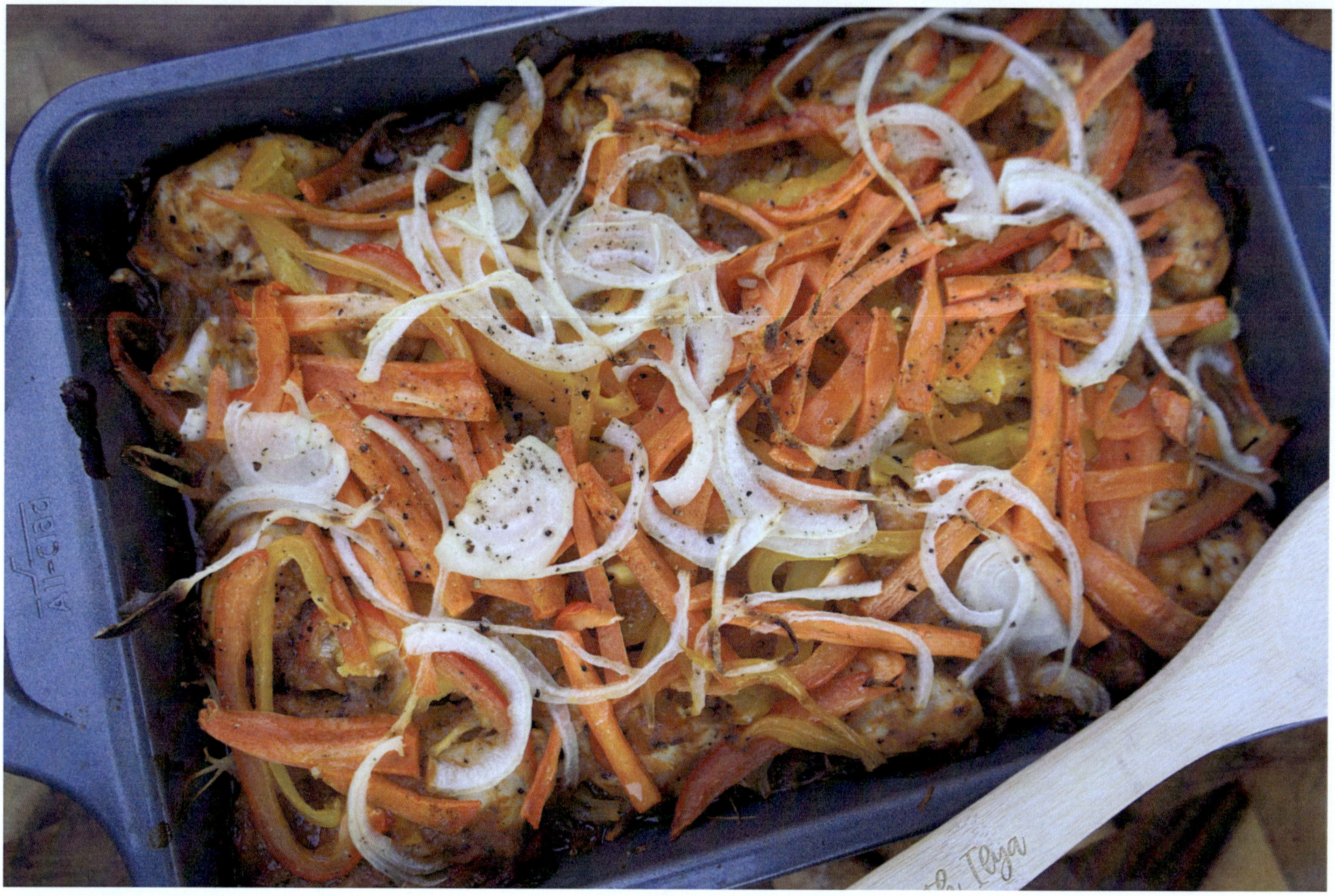

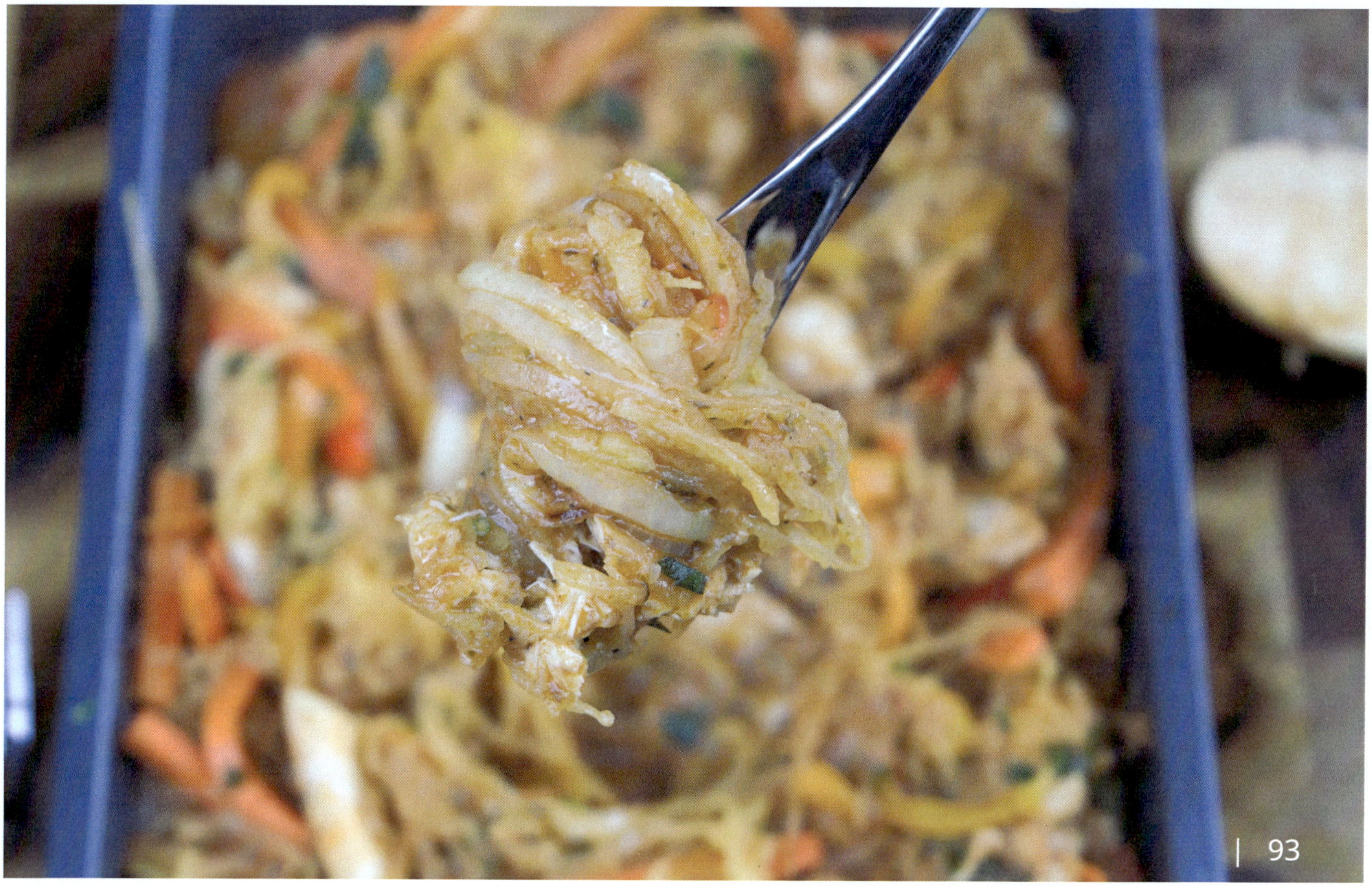

93

BUTTERNUT SQUASH WAFFLES

Turns out, you can make waffles out of almost anything! This time, I decided to try butternut squash, added chickpea flour for extra protein, and…surprisingly, it turned out pretty great. These waffles are savory, packed with protein, and perfect for brunch or a post-workout snack. This recipe makes 15 waffles.

Ingredients

- **1 medium butternut squash (poke holes and microwave for 15-20 minutes until soft)**
- **4 large eggs**
- **½ cup Greek yogurt**
- **1 cup shredded Gruyère cheese**
- **1 cup chickpea flour**
- **½ cup milk**
- **1 tsp baking powder**
- **Salt & pepper to taste**
- **1 tsp cinnamon powder**
- **Oil spray for waffle maker**
- **Toppings: arugula, burrata cheese, tomato slices, avocado slices, rock salt, balsamic glaze**

Instructions

- Cook the squash: microwave butternut squash for 15-20 minutes until soft. Slice in half, remove seeds, and scoop flesh into a bowl.
- Mix the batter: add eggs, Greek yogurt, Gruyère, chickpea flour, milk, baking powder, salt, and cinnamon. Mix until smooth.
- Cook the waffles: Preheat waffle maker, spray with oil, add batter (2-3 tbsp per waffle), and cook for 5 minutes until golden.
- Top & serve: garnish with arugula, burrata, tomatoes, avocado, rock salt, and balsamic glaze. Enjoy!

Scan to watch

Serves 5

Prep time 20 min

Cook time 15 min

Quick Tips:
- Let waffles cool on a wire rack instead of stacking them—this prevents sogginess.
- Cook extra waffles and freeze them. Reheat in a toaster for a quick, crispy breakfast.

Macros per Waffle: Calories: 71 | Protein: 4g | Carbs: 6g | Fat: 3g

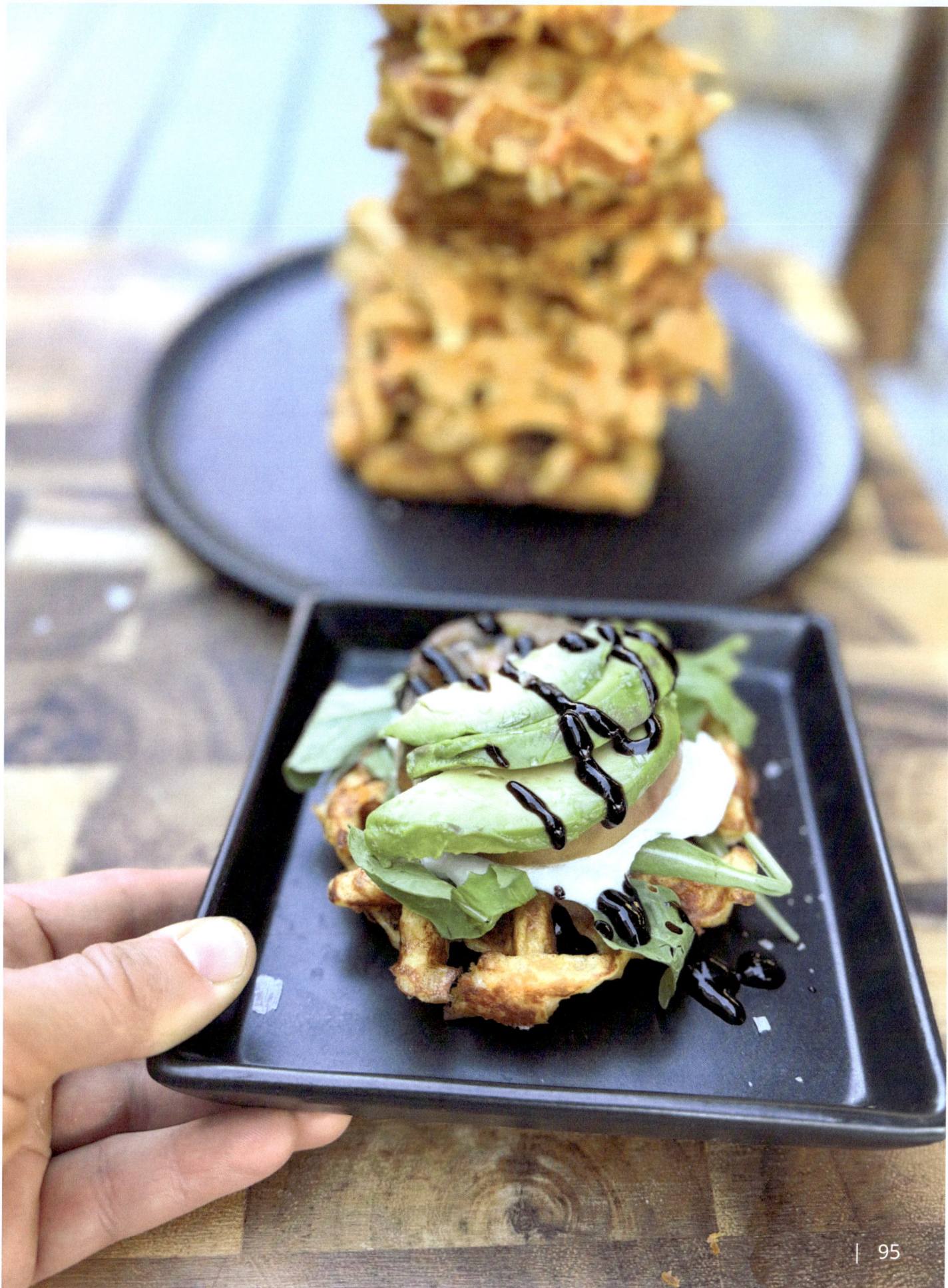

EVERYTHING-BUT-THE-FRIDGE CASSEROLE

Sometimes, the best meals come from sheer improvisation. This casserole is exactly that—a great cooking hack to clean up your fridge while making something delicious. Toss in whatever you have on hand, bake, and enjoy a cozy, satisfying dish.

Ingredients

- **4-5 slices cabbage**
- **6 Italian sausages (cooked on a skillet)**
- **2 cups mushrooms (sautéed with sausage)**
- **1 cup cherry tomatoes**
- **1 cup carrots, chopped**
- **1 cup ricotta cheese**
- **½ cup shredded Parmesan cheese**
- **½ cup shredded Gruyère cheese**
- **1 bell pepper, sliced**
- **1 red onion, sliced**
- **1 can (20 oz) tomato sauce**
- **Extra virgin olive oil**
- **Salt, pepper, garlic powder to taste**
- **Fresh basil leaves for topping**

Instructions

- Prep ingredients: cook the Italian sausage and mushrooms together in a skillet.
- Assemble: layer cabbage, cooked sausage, mushrooms, cherry tomatoes, carrots, ricotta, cheeses, bell pepper, and red onion in a large casserole dish.
- Season & add sauce: season with salt, pepper, and garlic powder. Pour tomato sauce over everything, then drizzle with olive oil.
- Bake: cover with foil and bake at 400°F for 40-50 minutes, or until everything is bubbling and fragrant.
- Top & serve: garnish with fresh basil and dig in!

Scan to watch

Serves 6

Prep time 15 min

Cook time 50 min

Quick Tips:
- Swap out ingredients based on what's in your fridge—leftover roasted veggies, different cheeses, or another protein all work.

Calories: 320 | Protein: 22g | Carbs: 18g | Fat: 18g

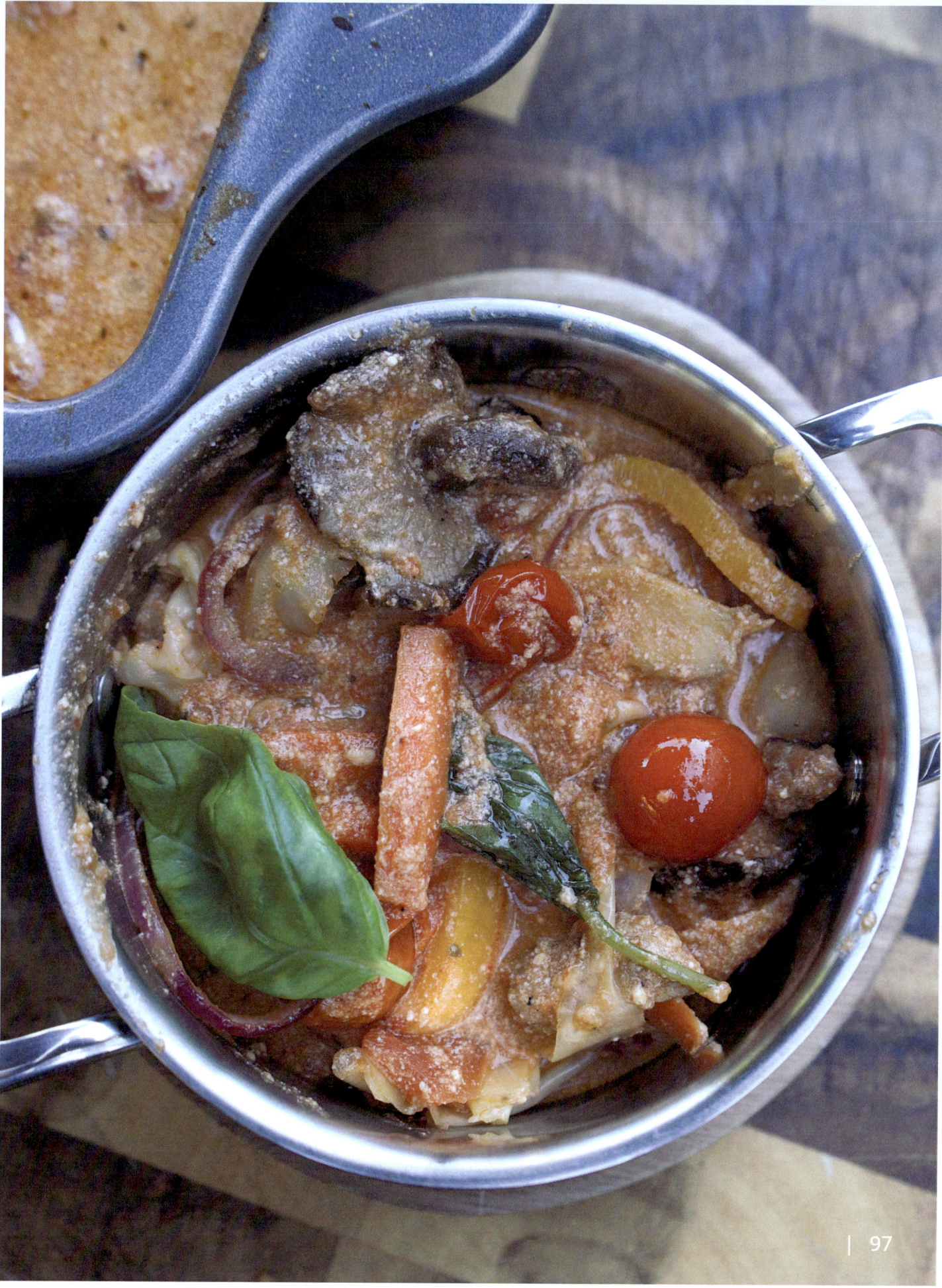

MEDITERRANEAN STYLE LENTIL BREAD

This bread is packed with protein and keeps the carbs to a minimum. It's the kind of recipe that makes your snack time or side dish feel like a win. Plus, it's super customizable depending on what you have on hand.

Ingredients

- **1 cup red lentils (soaked overnight)**
- **2 eggs**
- **½ cup Greek yogurt**
- **3 tbsp extra virgin olive oil**
- **½ cup parsley, chopped**
- **¼ cup olives, chopped**
- **¼ cup sun-dried tomatoes, chopped (optional)**
- **½ cup feta cheese**
- **1 tsp baking powder**
- **Salt & pepper to taste (add extra if omitting salty ingredients)**
- **¼ cup pumpkin seeds (optional, for topping)**

Instructions

- Prep the lentils: soak the red lentils overnight in 2 cups of water. Drain before using.
- Blend the base: add soaked lentils, eggs, yogurt, and olive oil to a blender. Blend until smooth.
- Mix it up: pour the mixture into a bowl. Stir in parsley, olives, sun-dried tomatoes, feta, baking powder, salt, and pepper.
- Bake: transfer to a parchment-lined baking dish. Sprinkle pumpkin seeds on top. Bake at 350°F for 45-55 minutes, or until firm and golden.
- Cool & slice: let it cool slightly before slicing. Enjoy warm or at room temperature. Serve with Hummus, avocado, or tzatziki

Scan to watch

Serves 8

Prep time
10 min

Cook time
50 min

Quick Tips:
- Mini muffins: pour into a muffin tin for grab-and-go protein bites. Reduce bake time to ~25 mins.
- Add grated carrot or zucchini to sneak in extra veg.

Calories: 120 | Protein: 8g | Carbs: 6g | Fat: 6g

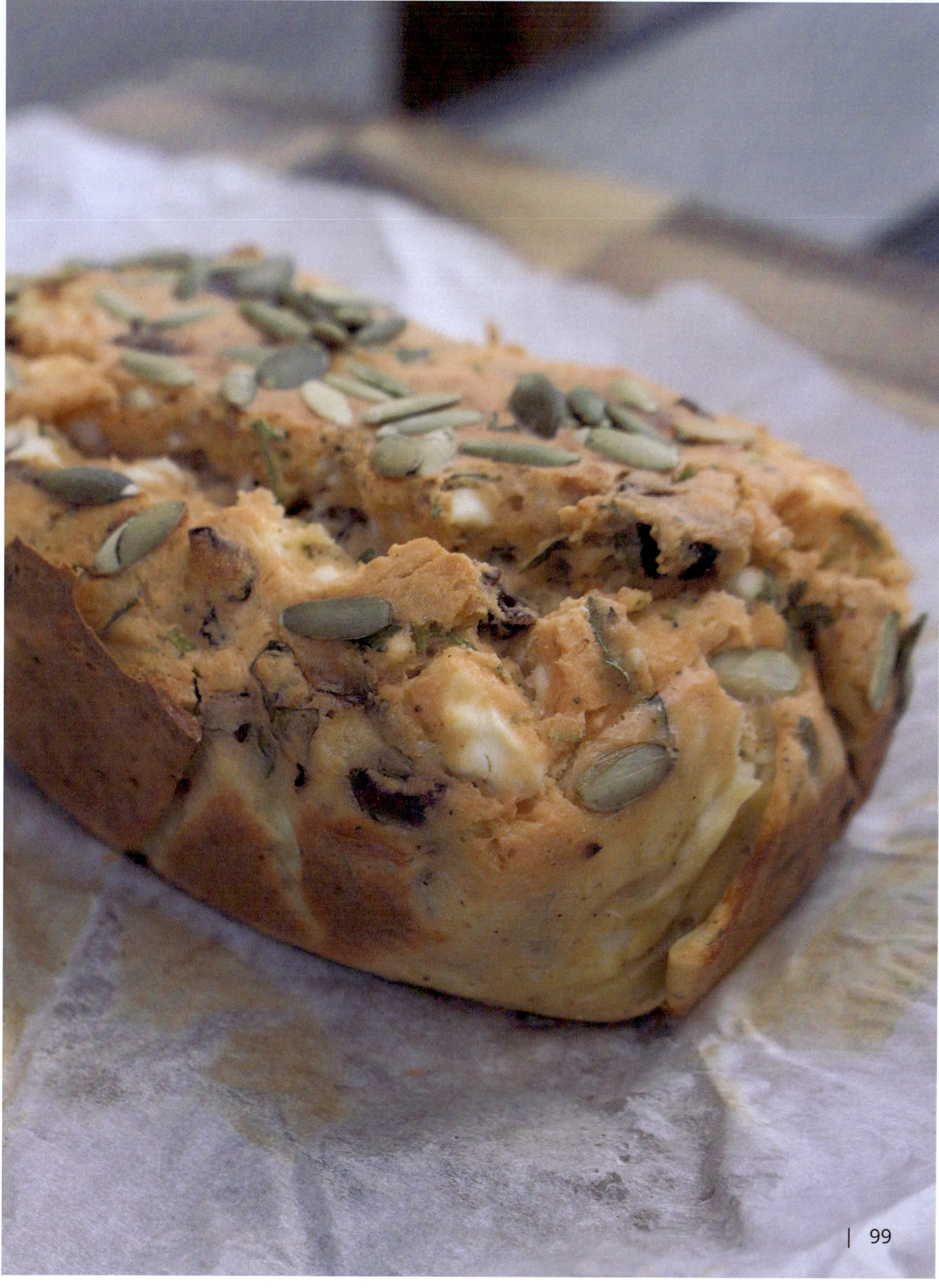

SHAWARMA CHICKEN

Flavor-packed and meal-prep friendly! These wraps are a total lunch or dinner win—customizable, satisfying, and full of Mediterranean flavor.

Ingredients

For the Chicken:
- 2 lb boneless skinless chicken thighs
- 1 cup Greek yogurt
- 3 tbsp olive oil
- 5 cloves garlic, minced
- 1/2 cup parsley, chopped
- Juice of 1 lemon
- 1 tbsp cumin, 1 tbsp coriander
- 2 tsp smoked paprika
- 1 tsp turmeric, 1 tsp cinnamon
- 1/2 tsp cayenne (optional), 1 tbsp salt, 1/2 tsp pepper
- 2 bell peppers, sliced
- 2 onions, thick-cut rings

For the Tzatziki:
- 1 cup Greek yogurt
- 1 cucumber (grated)
- 2 cloves garlic, minced
- 1 tbsp olive oil, 1 tbsp lemon juice
- 1 tbsp dill or mint, chopped
- Salt & pepper to taste

Instructions

- Marinate chicken: in a large bowl, mix yogurt, olive oil, garlic, parsley, lemon juice, cumin, coriander, smoked paprika, turmeric, cinnamon, cayenne, salt, and pepper. Add chicken thighs and coat well. Cover and marinate in the fridge for at least 1 hour.
- Air fry chicken: preheat air fryer to 375°F. Place thick onion rings flat in the air fryer basket to act as a base. Thread chicken and bell pepper slices onto skewers and stand them upright in the onion rings. Air fry for 15–20 minutes, turning once, until chicken is fully cooked and slightly charred. Chop chicken, peppers, and cooked onion rings into bite-sized pieces.
- Make tzatziki: combine Greek yogurt, grated cucumber (squeeze out moisture), garlic, olive oil, lemon juice, dill or mint, and salt and pepper. Mix well and chill until ready to use.

Scan to watch

Serves 4

Prep time 25 min

Cook time 25 min

Quick Tips:
- Add a quick Mediterranean salad (tomatoes, cukes, onions, parsley + olive oil + vinegar) and some crispy air fryer fries. Wrap it all up in lavash with lettuce and tzatziki for the ultimate combo!

Per Wrap: Calories: 420 | Protein: 29g | Carbs: 36g | Fat: 17g

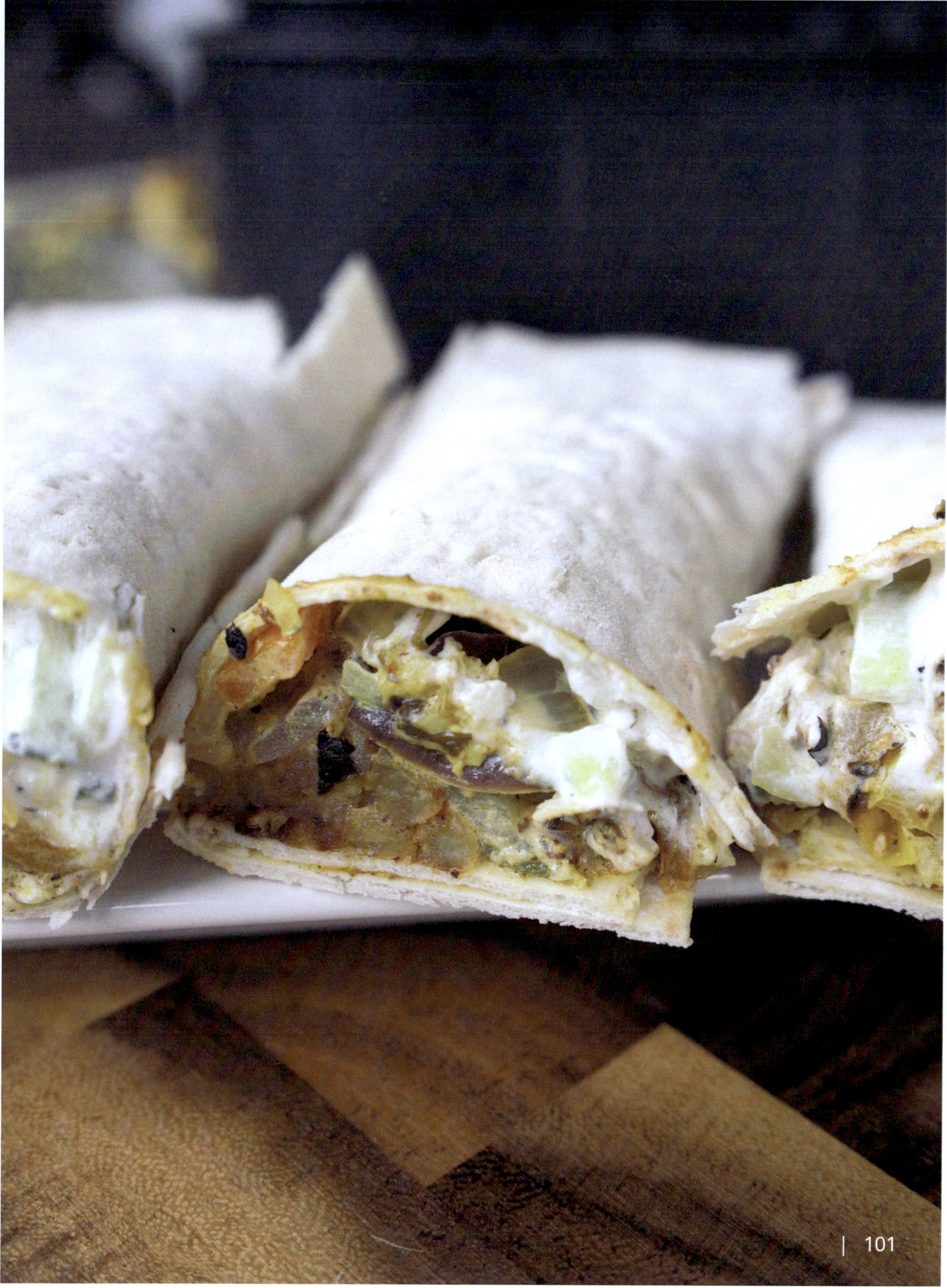

HONEY CHICKEN WITH POTATOES, APPLES & BRIE

Sweet, savory, and effortlessly elegant—this dish is dinner party gold. Everyone gets their own deliciously layered tray, and trust me, no one leaves unimpressed.

Ingredients

- **2 lbs chicken thighs (about 8)**
- **6 yellow potatoes, thinly sliced**
- **2 apples, thinly sliced**
- **2–3 tbsp olive oil**
- **1 1/2 tbsp fruit vinegar**
- **1 1/2 tbsp paprika**
- **Salt & pepper to taste**
- **Brie cheese, sliced (3 slices per serving)**
- **Fresh basil, for garnish**

For the Honey Sauce:

- **4 tbsp spicy or regular honey**
- **2 tbsp honey mustard**
- **1 tbsp olive oil**
- **1 tbsp fruit vinegar**
- **1 tsp garlic powder**
- **Salt & pepper to taste**
- **Fresh thyme (a few sprigs)**

Instructions

- Prep potatoes & apples: thinly slice potatoes and apples. In a bowl, toss potato slices with olive oil, vinegar, paprika, salt, and pepper. Set apples aside.
- Make sauce: combine all honey sauce ingredients in a bowl. Split into two parts: one for baking, one for serving.
- Assemble individual trays: cut foil squares and fold up the edges to form 8 mini trays. In each tray, layer potatoes, apples, 3 slices of brie, and top with a chicken thigh. Brush chicken with half the honey sauce.
- Bake: place trays on a baking sheet. Bake at 375°F for 30–35 minutes, until chicken reaches 165°F and potatoes are tender.
- Finish & serve: drizzle with remaining honey sauce, garnish with fresh basil, and serve hot.

Scan to watch

Serves 8

Prep time 20 min

Cook time 35 min

Quick Tips:

- Make-ahead tip: prep the trays ahead of time, cover with foil, and refrigerate for up to 24 hours. When you're ready, bake them straight from the fridge—perfect for entertaining!

Calories: 360 | Protein: 26g | Carbs: 25g | Fat: 18g

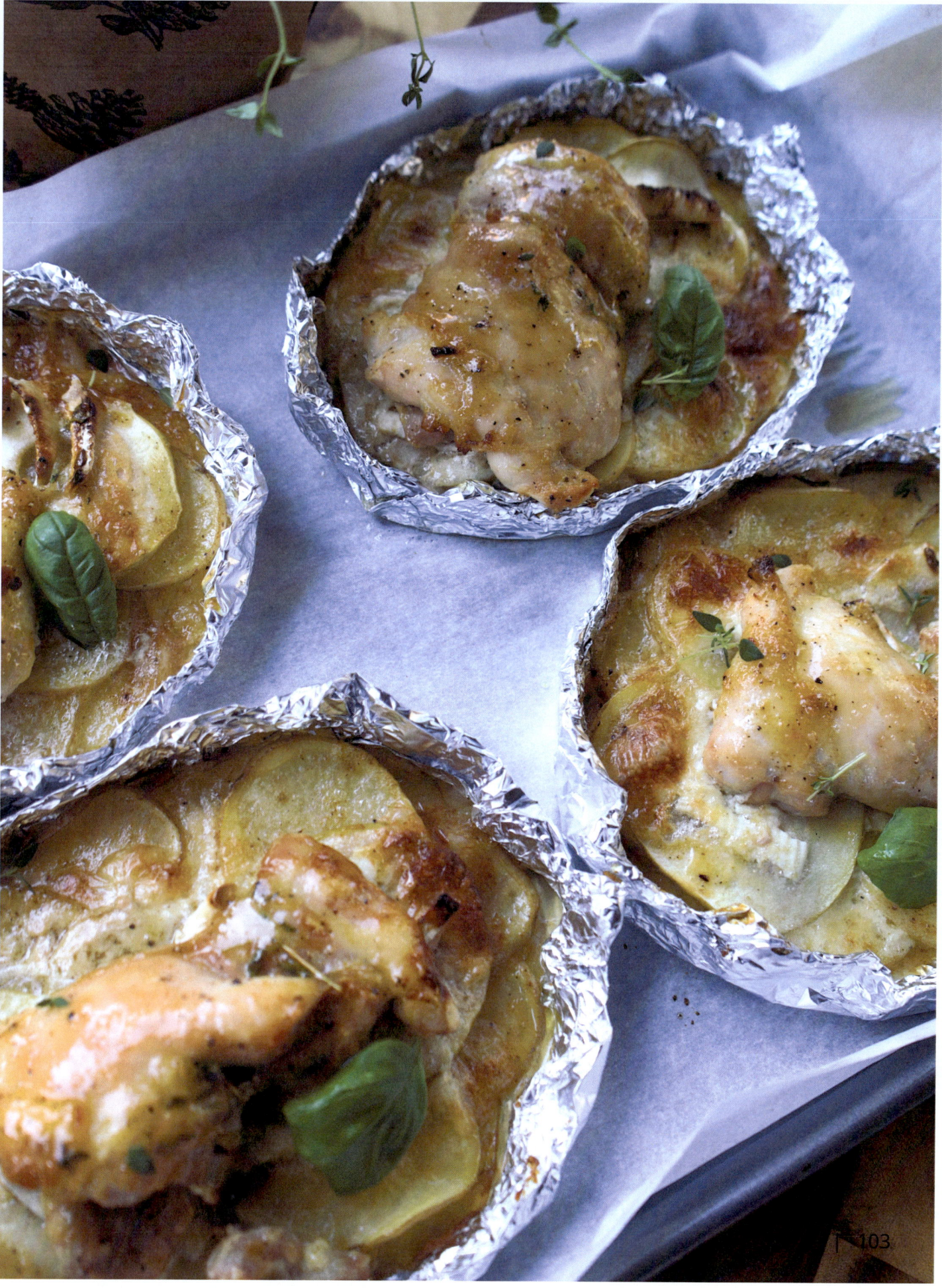

PANKO-CRUSTED CHICKEN

This recipe started as a friend's suggestion, but it quickly became a weeknight favorite. Crispy panko chicken pairs with a creamy pesto and veggie mix that feels fancy but is secretly fuss-free.

Ingredients

Air-Fried Panko Chicken:
- 10 chicken tenders
- 1½ cups flour, salt & pepper
- 2 large eggs, beaten
- 1½ cups panko breadcrumbs
- Oil spray

Pistachio Pesto:
- ½ cup pistachios
- ½ cup basil
- Juice of 1 lemon
- 2 tbsp olive oil
- 2 garlic cloves
- ½ cup grated Parmesan
- Water, salt & pepper

Tomato-Mushroom-Bean Mix:
- ½ onion, chopped
- 3 garlic cloves, minced
- 2 cups cherry tomatoes
- 4 cups mushrooms
- 2 cans lima beans
- 1 tbsp tomato paste
- 3 tbsp Greek yogurt
- Cumin, Italian seasoning, salt & pepper

Instructions

- Preheat air fryer to 400°F. Set up a dredging station: flour with salt and pepper, beaten eggs, and panko in separate bowls. Coat chicken tenders in flour, egg, then panko. Spray lightly with oil and air fry 10–12 minutes, flipping halfway, until golden.
- In a food processor, blend pistachios, basil, lemon juice, olive oil, garlic, and Parmesan. Add water slowly to get a drizzle-worthy consistency. Season to taste.
- In a large skillet, sauté onion and garlic until soft. Add cherry tomatoes and cook until they begin to burst. Stir in mushrooms, beans, tomato paste, sour cream, and seasoning. Simmer for 5–6 minutes until thick and flavorful.
- Plate the chicken with a scoop of the veggie-bean mix. Drizzle with pesto.

Scan to watch

Serves 10

Prep time 25 min

Cook time 20 min

Quick Tips:
- Swap pistachios for walnuts or almonds in the pesto.
- Use white beans or chickpeas if lima beans aren't your thing.
- Chicken still not crispy? Give it another 2 minutes in the air fryer.

Calories: 320 | Protein: 28g | Carbs: 22g | Fat: 14g

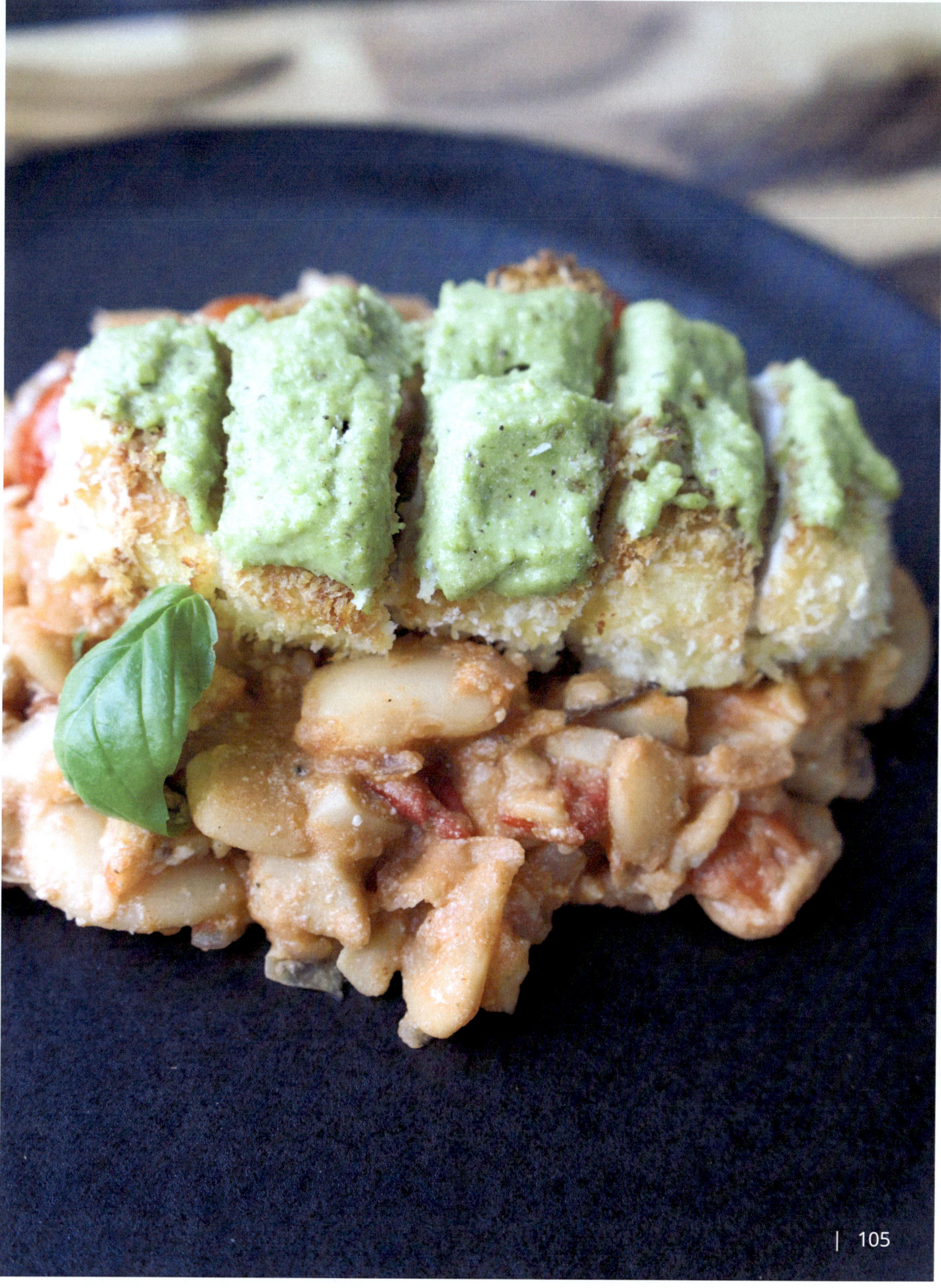

STUFFED BAKED POTATO WITH SHREDDED CHICKEN

This recipe came from my deep devotion to anything stuffed, loaded, and unapologetically satisfying. If your baked potato isn't a full meal, are you even trying?

Ingredients

- **1 medium russet potato, scrubbed and rinsed**
- **1 oz Brie cheese (or Boursin), sliced**
- **1 oz shredded Gruyère cheese**
- **Salt and pepper, to taste**
- **Oil spray**
- **4–5 cherry tomatoes, sliced**
- **¼ bell pepper, sliced**
- **1 green scallion, chopped**
- **1 chicken tenderloin**
- **1 tbsp sriracha**
- **2 tbsp pepita salsa (or any salsa you like)**
- **Toppings: sour cream, chopped scallions, and that leftover salsa from the Instant Pot**

Instructions

- Place the potato on a trivet in the Instant Pot with 1 cup of water. Pressure cook on High for 10 minutes. Let pressure release naturally.
- Add the chicken tenderloin, salsa, sriracha, salt, and pepper to the Instant Pot. Pressure cook on High for 30 minutes. Do a quick release and shred the chicken with two forks. Keep any leftover liquid—it's gold.
- Slice open the baked potato. Season with salt and pepper, then stuff with sliced Brie and Gruyère. Pile on the shredded chicken, tomatoes, bell pepper, and scallions. Spray with oil. Bake at 400°F for 10 minutes or until the cheese is melted and bubbly.
- Finish with Toppings
- Top with sour cream, extra scallions, and that leftover salsa sauce from the chicken.

Scan to watch

Serves 1

Prep time 10 min

Cook time 40 min

Quick Tips:
- Leftovers? Double the chicken and save it for wraps or bowls tomorrow.
- Save time by using leftover rotisserie chicken!

Calories: 380 | Protein: 20g | Carbs: 30g | Fat: 20g

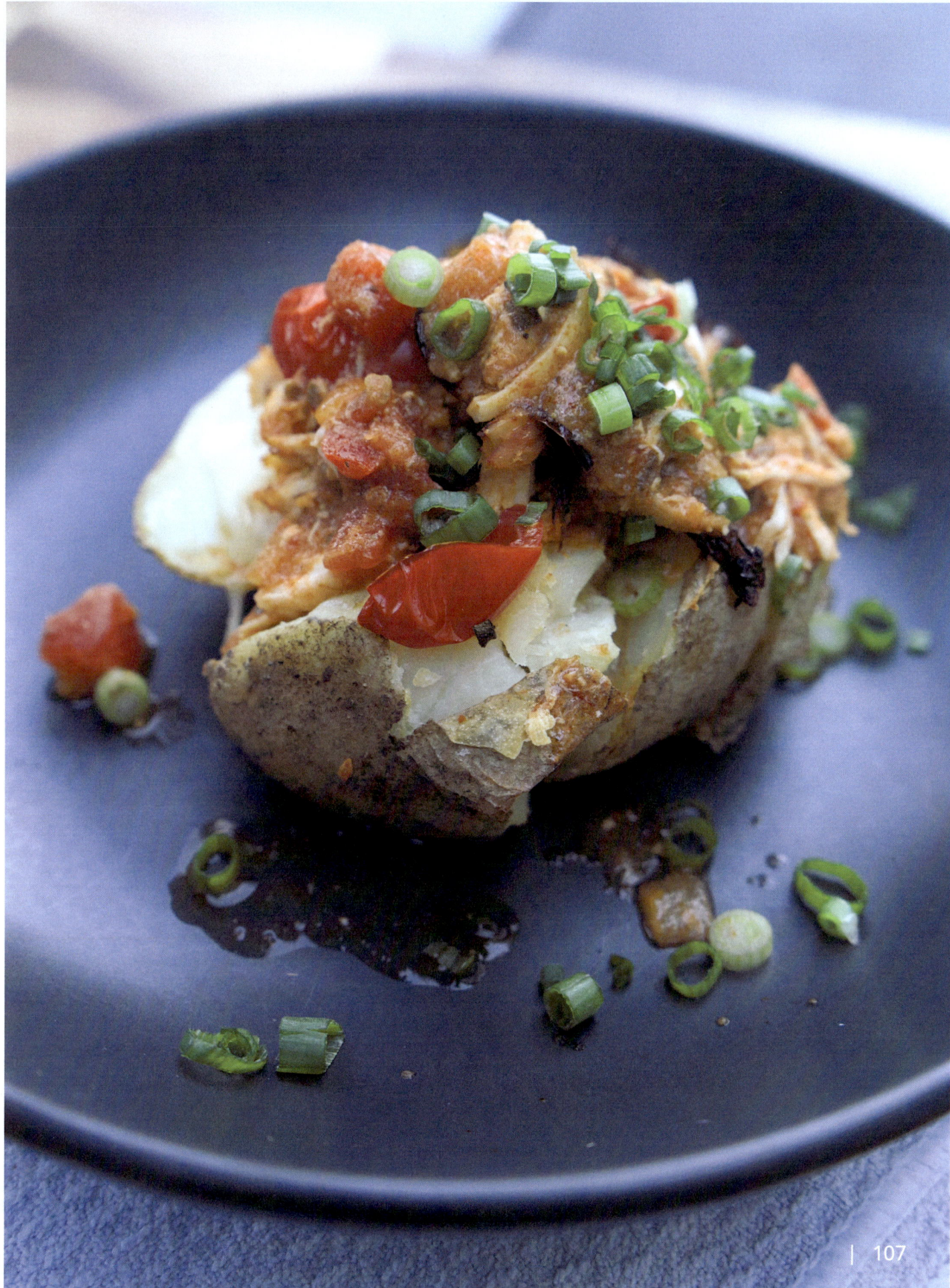

WHOOPS, ENCHILADA CASSEROLE

Sometimes the best recipes come from happy accidents! What started as an attempt to make stuffed pizza pockets ended up as this high-protein, low-carb casserole that's packed with flavor and comfort—no stuffing required!

Ingredients

For the Meat Filling:
- 1 onion, chopped
- 4 garlic cloves, minced
- 1 lb ground beef
- 1 can diced tomatoes
- 2 tbsp red chili paste
- Salt, pepper, cumin, paprika, chili powder (to taste)
- 1 cup parsley, chopped
- 1 can black beans, drained

For the Casserole:
- Fajita or enchilada sauce
- 12 low-carb tortillas
- 2 cups shredded cheese (Gruyere & Mexican blend for extra gooeyness)

For Toppings: enchilada or fajitas sauce, sriracha sauce, avocado slices, jalapenos, cilantro, sour cream

Instructions

- Make the meat filling: sauté chopped onion until soft, then add minced garlic. Add ground beef and cook halfway. Stir in diced tomatoes, chili paste, black beans, parsley, and spices. Cook until beef is fully browned.
- Layer the casserole: spread a layer of sauce in the bottom of a baking dish. Layer tortillas, meat filling, and cheese. Repeat the layers (tortillas, meat, cheese) three times, ending with cheese on top.
- Bake it up: preheat oven or air fryer to 375°F. Cover with foil and bake for 20 minutes. Remove foil halfway to let cheese bubble and brown.
- Top and serve: garnish with sauce, sriracha, avocado, jalapenos, cilantro, and sour cream.

Scan to watch

Serves 5

Prep time 20 min

Cook time 25 min

Quick Tips:
- Use your favorite enchilada sauce for a more traditional flavor!
- Add crunchy tortilla chips on top for texture.
- This casserole tastes even better the next day—perfect for meal prep!

Calories: ~400 | Protein: 25g | Carbs: 20g | Fat: 24g

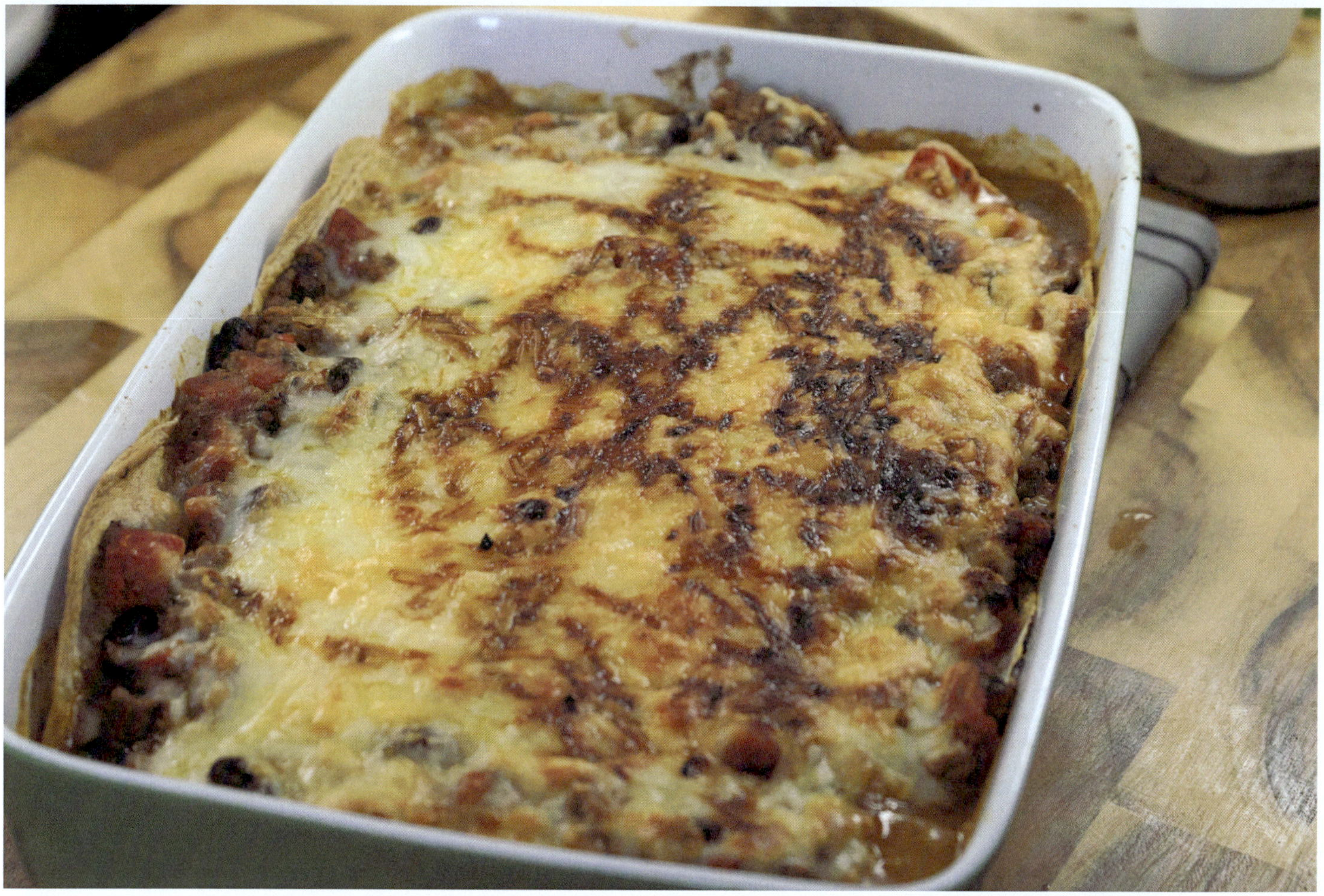

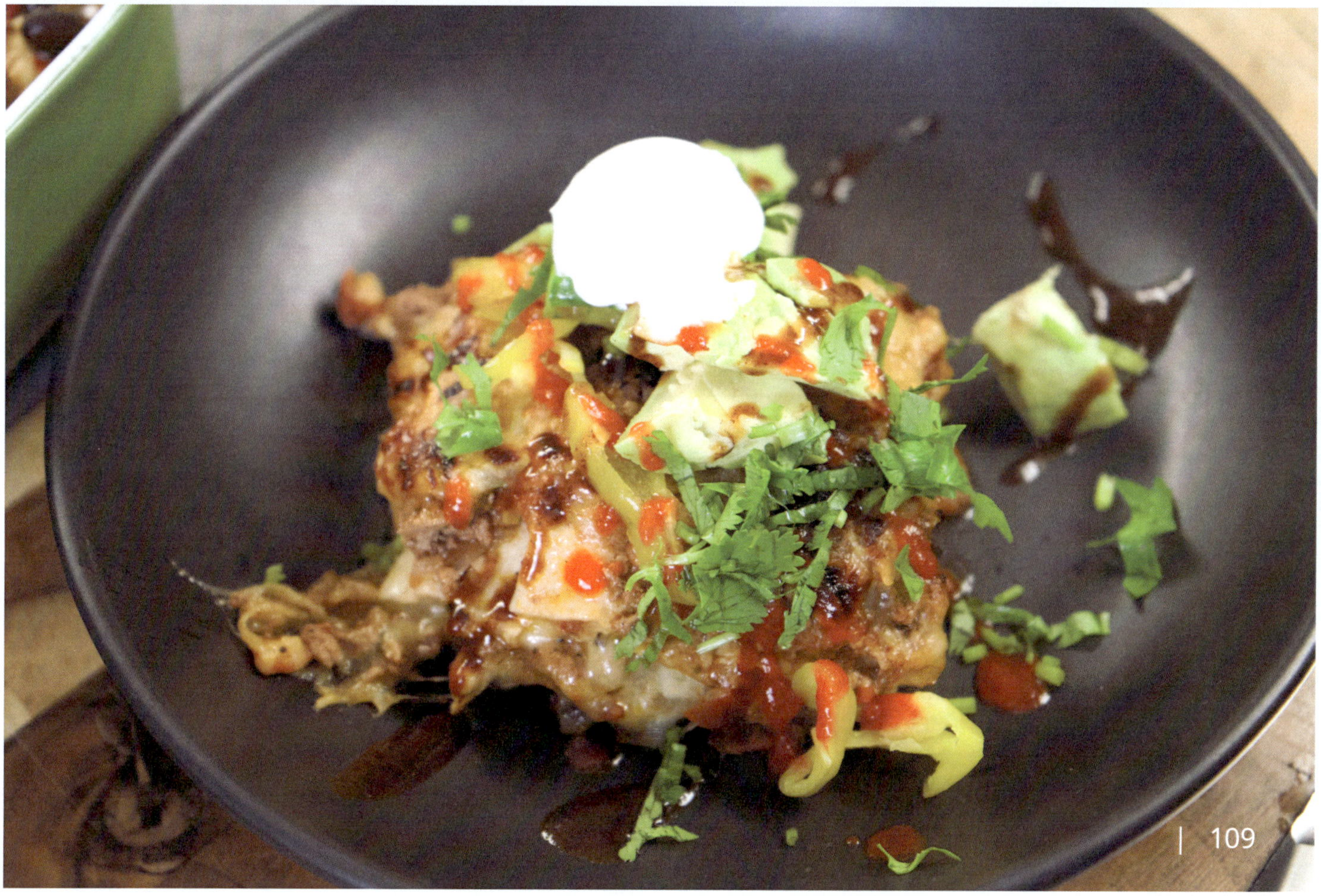

109

PICKLED BRINE + FETA WHOLE CHICKEN

If you love pickled flavors, this one's going to ruin plain roast chicken for you forever. Marinating a whole chicken in pickle brine and feta gives you insane flavor and the juiciest bird ever. Roasting it over seasoned potatoes? Just showing off at this point.

Ingredients

For the Chicken:
- 1 whole chicken
- 1 cup pickle brine (from the jar)
- 2–3 pickled cucumbers (optional)
- ½ cup crumbled feta
- Oil spray
- Salt & pepper to taste

For the Roasted Potatoes:
- 10 yellow potatoes
- Salt, pepper, paprika, garlic powder
- Oil spray
- 1 jalapeño, sliced
- ⅓ cup chopped parsley
- ⅓ cup chopped dill
- ⅓ cup chopped scallions
- 5 pickles, chopped
- 1 cup crumbled feta
- Juice of 1 lemon
- 1 tomato, chopped
- 2 tbsp extra virgin olive oil
- 1 tbsp fruit vinegar

Instructions

- Blend feta, pickles, and pickle brine until smooth. Smother the chicken all over. Cover and refrigerate for at least 4 hours.
- Quarter potatoes, season with salt, pepper, paprika, and garlic powder, and spray lightly with oil.
- Preheat oven or air fryer to 375°F. Arrange potatoes in a roasting tray. Place the marinated chicken on a rack above the potatoes. Spray chicken with oil, season with salt and pepper, and roast for about 1 hour, flipping halfway through for extra crispy skin. Chicken is done when it hits 165°F internally.
- Toss the roasted potatoes with jalapeños, parsley, dill, scallions, chopped pickles, crumbled feta, lemon juice, tomatoes, olive oil, and fruit vinegar.

Scan to watch

Serves 6

Prep time 10 min + marinating

Cook time 60 min

Quick Tips:
- Marinate for just 1 hour at room temp if you forget to do it the night before.
- Pat the chicken dry before roasting and only lightly spray with oil.
- Make broth or soup with the leftover chicken bones.

Calories: 510 | Protein: 42g | Carbs: 29g | Fat: 27g

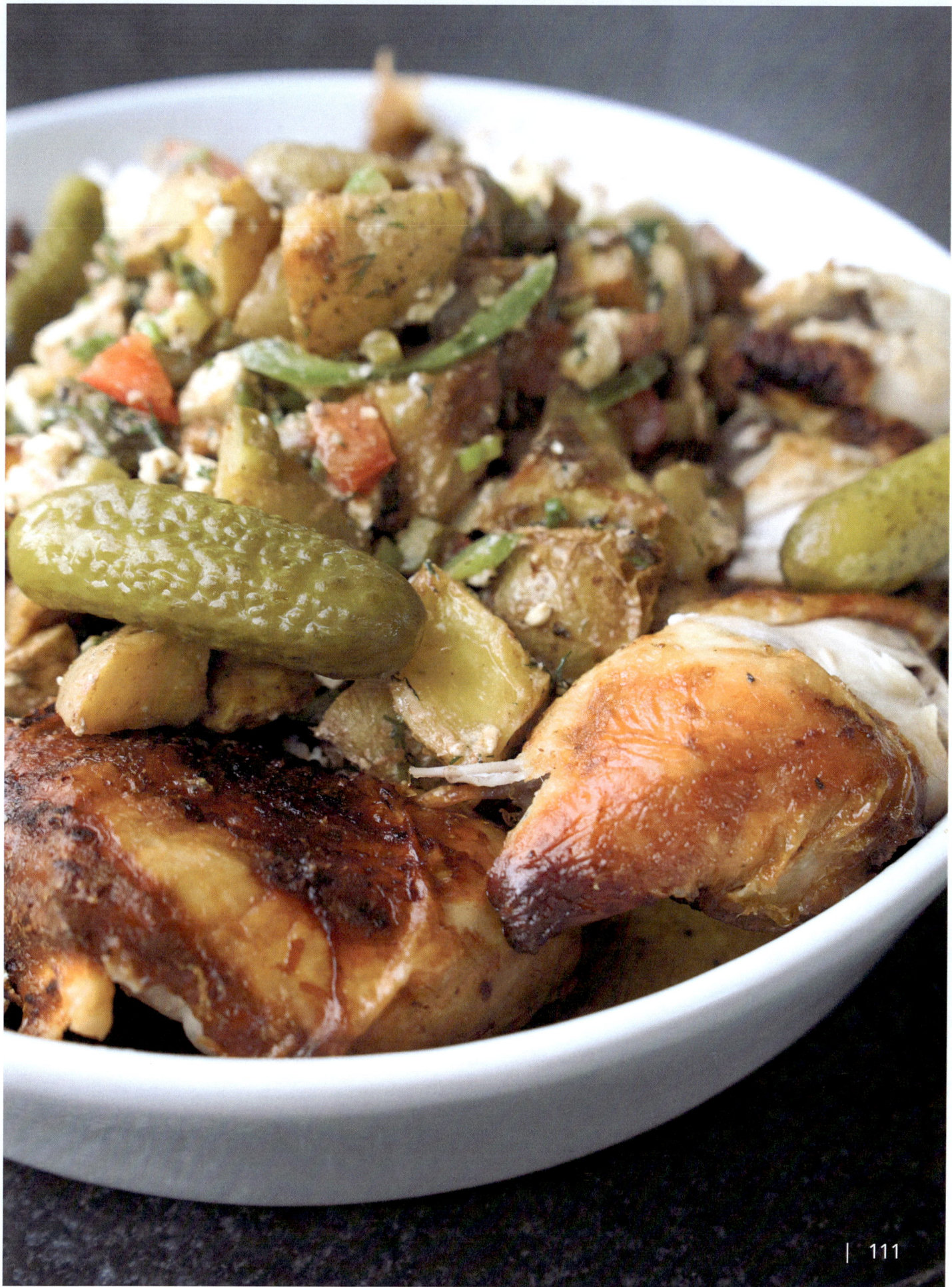

PEAR-FECTLY FRUITY CHICKEN SALAD

Strange combo? Maybe. Delicious? Absolutely. This protein-packed, low-carb wonder is the multitasking lunch or dinner salad your taste buds didn't even know they were waiting for.

Ingredients

For the Salad:
- ½ red onion, thinly sliced
- 4–5 cups arugula
- 2 cans chicken, drained
- ½ cup dried cranberries
- ½ cup walnuts
- 3 pears, thinly sliced and lightly grilled with a touch of oil
- 1 cup crumbled feta (or swap with goat cheese or ricotta)

For the Vinaigrette:
- 3½ tbsp extra virgin olive oil
- 1½ tbsp balsamic vinegar
- 1 tbsp Dijon mustard
- 1 tsp garlic paste
- Salt & pepper to taste
- 1 tbsp honey

Instructions

- Toss walnuts in a dry skillet over medium heat until golden and fragrant.
- Drizzle oil in a skillet, add sliced pears, and grill for 2 minutes per side until caramelized.
- Layer arugula, chicken, red onion, cranberries, grilled pears, walnuts, and feta.
- In a jar, combine olive oil, balsamic vinegar, Dijon, garlic paste, honey, salt, and pepper. Shake it like you're mixing a cocktail.
- Drizzle vinaigrette over the salad, toss lightly, and get ready to enjoy.

Scan to watch

Serves 3

Prep time
15 min

Cook time
5 min

Quick Tips:
- Swap canned chicken for rotisserie or grilled thighs.
- Double the dressing and keep it in the fridge — it's killer over roasted veggies too.

Calories: ~420 | Protein: ~35g | Carbs: ~18g | Fat: ~25g

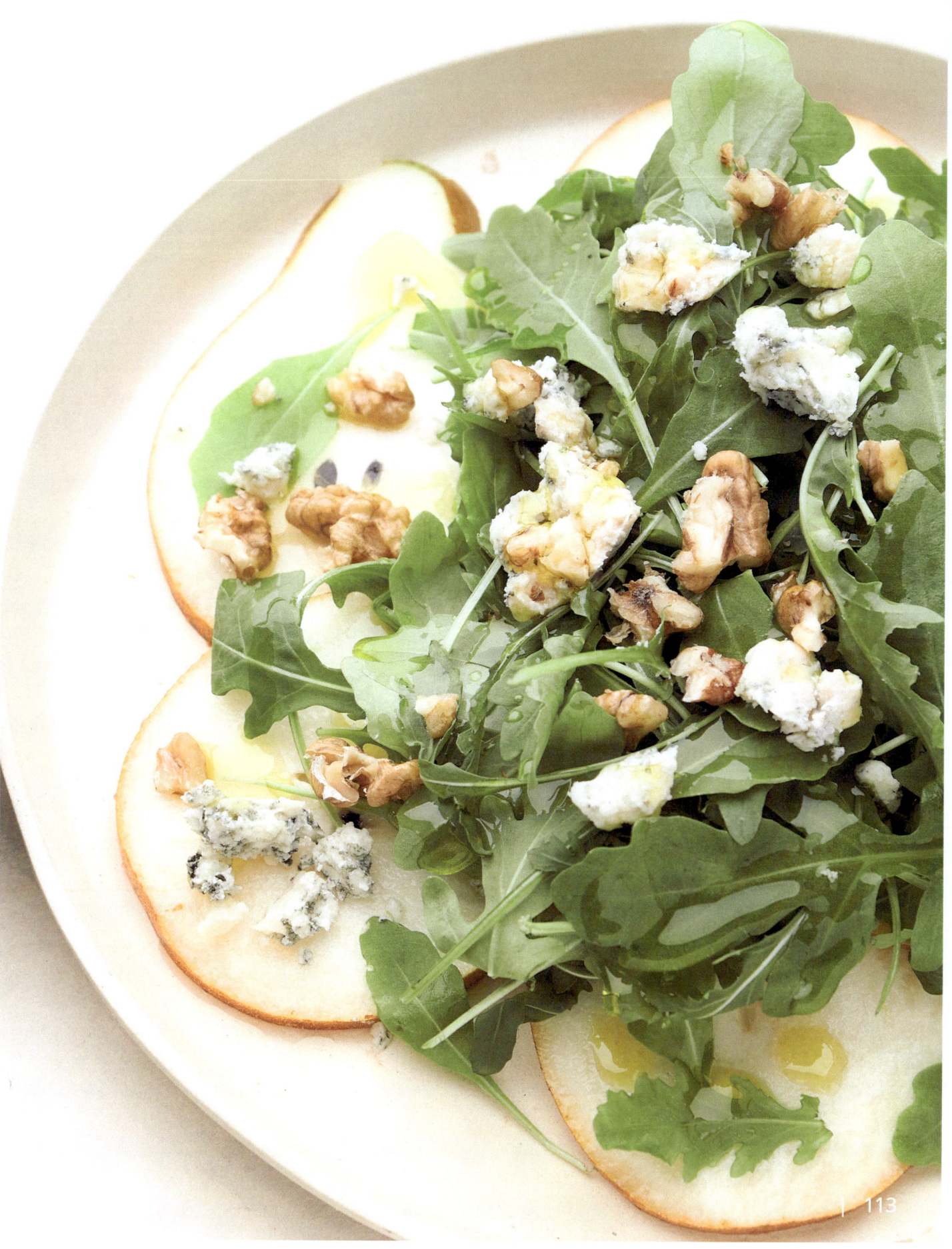

LAZY CAMPER'S SKILLET LASAGNA

Pasta, meat, cheese… and exactly one pan. Whether you're deep in the woods or just deep in your couch cushions, this lazy lasagna brings the comfort without the chaos.

Ingredients

- **Olive oil for sautéing**
- **1 onion, chopped**
- **4 cloves garlic, minced**
- **1 lb ground beef**
- **Salt and pepper to taste**
- **1 can (28 oz) San Marzano tomatoes**
- **1 can (14.5 oz) diced tomatoes**
- **1 tsp chili pepper powder**
- **1 cup water (plus more as needed)**
- **1 pack Trader Joe's lasagna noodles, broken into rustic, lazy chunks**
- **1 cup shredded Gruyere cheese**
- **1 ball burrata cheese**
- **Fresh basil — for garnish**

Instructions

- Sauté onion and garlic in olive oil until fragrant.
- Add beef, season, and brown; drain fat if needed.
- Stir in tomatoes, chili powder, and water; break up the tomatoes.
- Nestle broken noodles into sauce; simmer covered for 15–20 minutes, stirring occasionally. Add water if it gets thick.
- Top with Gruyere and burrata; cover for 2–3 minutes until melted.
- Garnish with basil and serve hot, straight from the skillet.

Scan to watch

Serves 4

Prep time
10 min

Cook time
30 min

Quick Tips:
- Using a heavy-bottomed skillet (like cast iron) distributes heat better and prevents burnt noodles.
- Throw a handful of spinach into the sauce for bonus nutrients.

Calories: ~520 | Protein: ~38g | Carbs: ~42g | Fat: ~28g

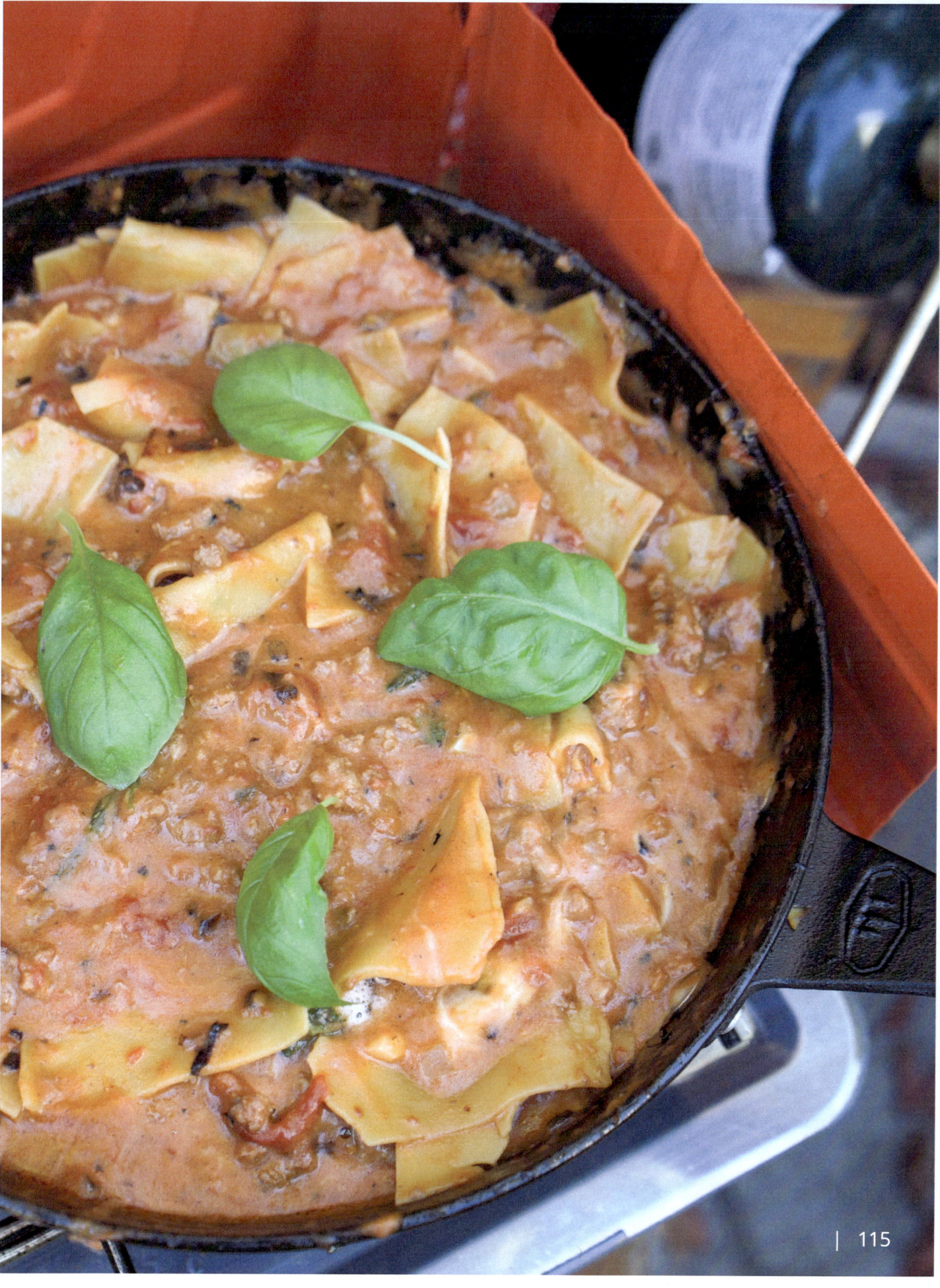

CABBAGE ROLLS (GOLYBCY, GALABKI)

Low-carb. High-protein. Freezer-friendly. Comfort food that feels like a hug without wrecking your macros. Crush four at a time, no regrets. Leftovers? Even better the next day (or next month from the freezer). Makes 32 rolls.

Ingredients

- 1 large cabbage head
- 2 lbs ground beef
- 2 ½ cups rice, parboiled
- 1 cup parsley, chopped
- 6 cloves garlic, minced
- 1 large onion, chopped
- 2 tsp each: salt, pepper, paprika, cumin
- 3–4 tbsp olive oil
- ½ cup tomato paste

For the Sauce:

- 1 onion, chopped
- 5 cloves garlic, minced
- 1 cup tomato paste
- 1 can (14 oz) diced tomatoes
- 1 can (28 oz) San Marzano tomatoes
- Salt, pepper, Italian seasoning to taste
- Oil for sautéing
- Hot water enough to cover rolls

Instructions

- Boil a large pot of water. Core the cabbage, peel leaves carefully, and blanch them for 2–3 minutes until flexible. Drain and cool. If stems are thick, shave them down to flatten.
- In a big bowl, mix ground beef, parboiled rice, parsley, garlic, onion, seasonings, olive oil, and tomato paste.
- Lay out a cabbage leaf, add about 2 tbsp of filling at the base, fold sides in, and roll tightly like a burrito.
- Simmer the sauce: In a large pot, sauté onion and garlic in oil. Stir in tomato paste, diced tomatoes, San Marzano tomatoes, and seasonings. Simmer for 10 minutes.
- Assemble & cook: nestle cabbage rolls into the sauce, add enough hot water to cover, and simmer on low for 1 hour.

Scan to watch

32 Rolls

Prep time 40 min

Cook time 60 min

Quick Tips:
- Frying the rolls briefly before simmering locks in extra flavor.
- Cabbage rolls freeze beautifully—stack them between parchment sheets.
- Don't forget the sour cream and a hit of fresh dill before serving.
- Add sautéed mushrooms to lighten the filling and boost umami. Great for stretching the meat.

Calories (per roll): ~85 | Protein: ~7g | Carbs: ~8g | Fat: ~4g

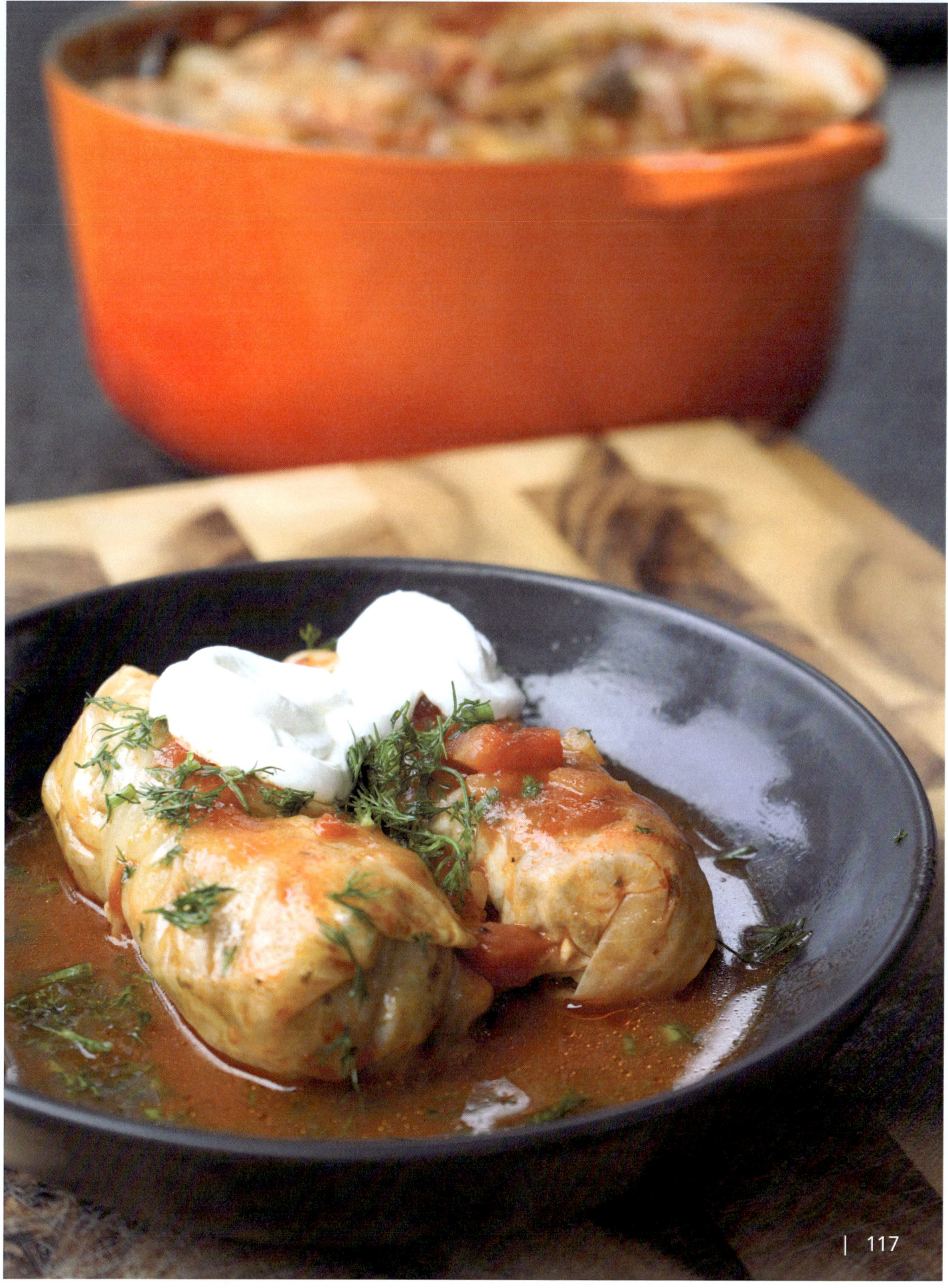

PROTEIN-PACKED RATATOUILLE

Cozy, hearty, and surprisingly filling—this ratatouille makes an easy main dish or a colorful Thanksgiving side. I love it with creamy polenta for the full fall comfort effect.

Ingredients

- **1 onion, chopped**
- **4 cloves garlic, minced**
- **2 eggplants, cubed**
- **1 jalapeño, chopped**
- **1 bell pepper, chopped**
- **2 zucchinis, cubed**
- **2 cans beans, drained (pinto and white work great)**
- **4 Argentinian sausages, sliced**
- **1 can diced tomatoes (14 oz)**
- **1 can San Marzano tomatoes (28 oz)**
- **Salt, pepper, thyme, sage, cumin to taste**
- **Fresh basil for topping**
- **Olive oil for sautéing**
- **Cooked polenta for serving (optional)**

Instructions

- In a large pot, heat olive oil. Cook onion until translucent, then add garlic and sauté until fragrant.
- Add cubed eggplant and cook for about 10 minutes, stirring occasionally.
- Stir in jalapeño, bell pepper, and zucchini. Cook for another 5 minutes.
- Mix in sliced sausages and drained beans. Let everything heat through.
- Pour in both cans of tomatoes. Season generously with salt, pepper, thyme, sage, and cumin.
- Cover and simmer on low heat for 30 minutes, stirring occasionally.
- Top with fresh basil. Serve warm with creamy polenta.

Scan to watch

Serves 10

Prep time
20 min

Cook time
45 min

Quick Tips:
- Perfect for meal prep or holiday dinners.
- Use chickpeas, kidney beans, black beans, or whatever you have lurking in the pantry.
- Not a sausage fan? Swap in shredded chicken or turkey.

Calories: ~320 | Protein: ~20g | Carbs: ~28g | Fat: ~12g

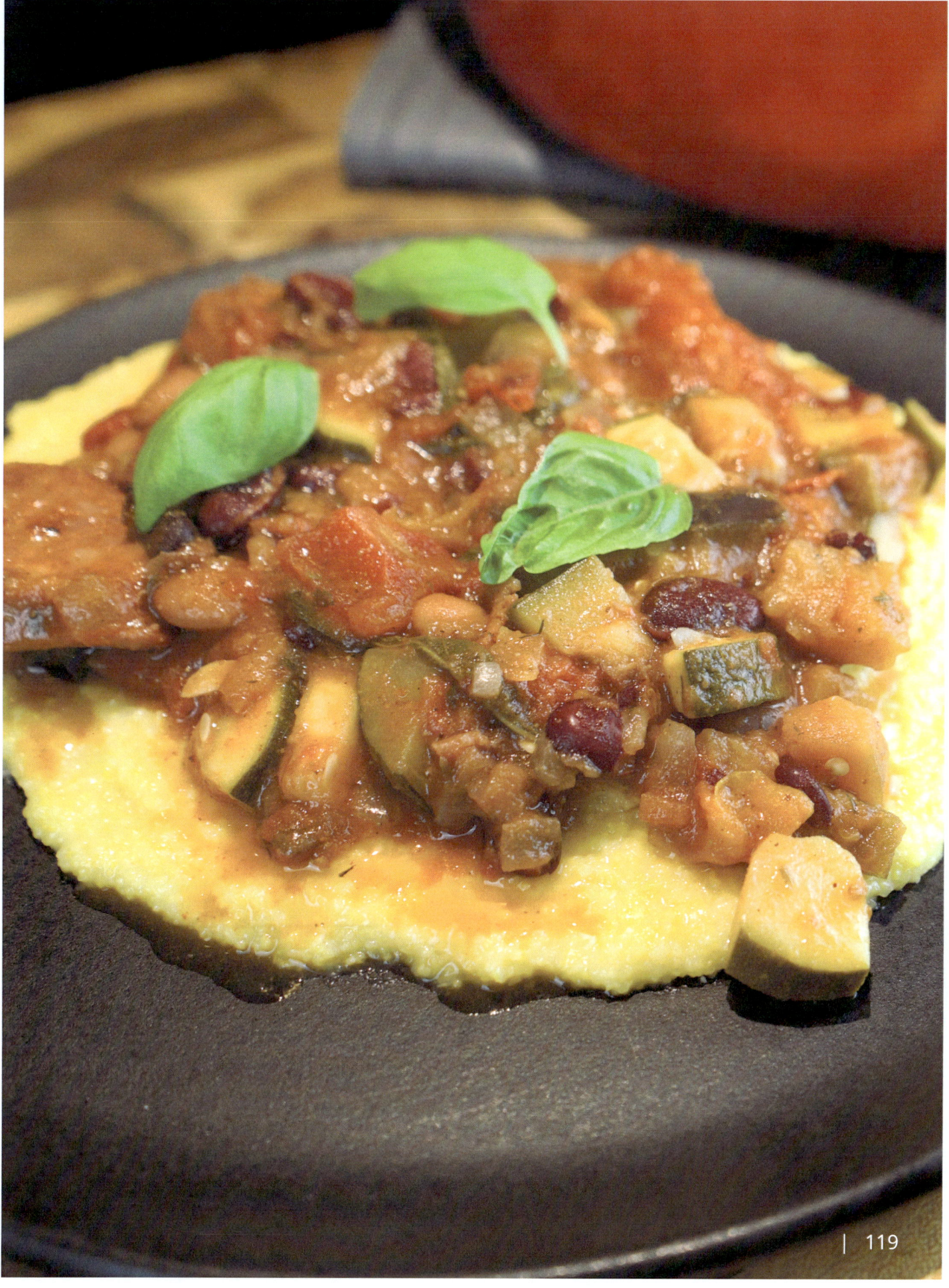

LEFTOVER TURKEY MASHED POTATO CRUNCH BALLS

You could reheat your Thanksgiving leftovers like a rookie… or you could roll them into crispy, golden bliss bombs instead. These crunch balls are low-carb, high-protein, and frankly? Possibly better than Thanksgiving dinner itself.

Ingredients

- **2 cups cooked turkey, shredded**
- **4 cups mashed potatoes**
- **1 cup cranberry sauce**
- **1 cup shredded cheese, any kind you love**
- **2 eggs, beaten**
- **2 cups panko crumbs**
- **Oil spray for crisping**

Instructions

- Use a large scoop (about 2 tablespoons) of mashed potatoes. Press it against the scoop sides to create a little cavity.
- Fill with shredded turkey, cranberry sauce, and cheese. Seal it with a little more mashed potato and gently shape into a ball.
- Dip each ball in beaten eggs, then roll in panko crumbs. Spray lightly with oil.
- Air fry at 380°F for 22–25 minutes, flipping halfway through. No air fryer? Pan-fry in a little oil until golden brown and crispy.
- Let them cool slightly and enjoy immediately!

Scan to watch

15 balls

Prep time
10 min

Cook time
25 min

Quick Tips:
- Swap turkey for ham, roast chicken, or even green bean casserole.
- Shape the balls, coat them in panko, and freeze uncooked. Bake straight from frozen at 400°F for 30–35 minutes.
- Pair with leftover gravy, ranch dip, or a spicy aioli.

Calories (per ball): ~150 | Protein: ~9g | Carbs: ~12g | Fat: ~6g

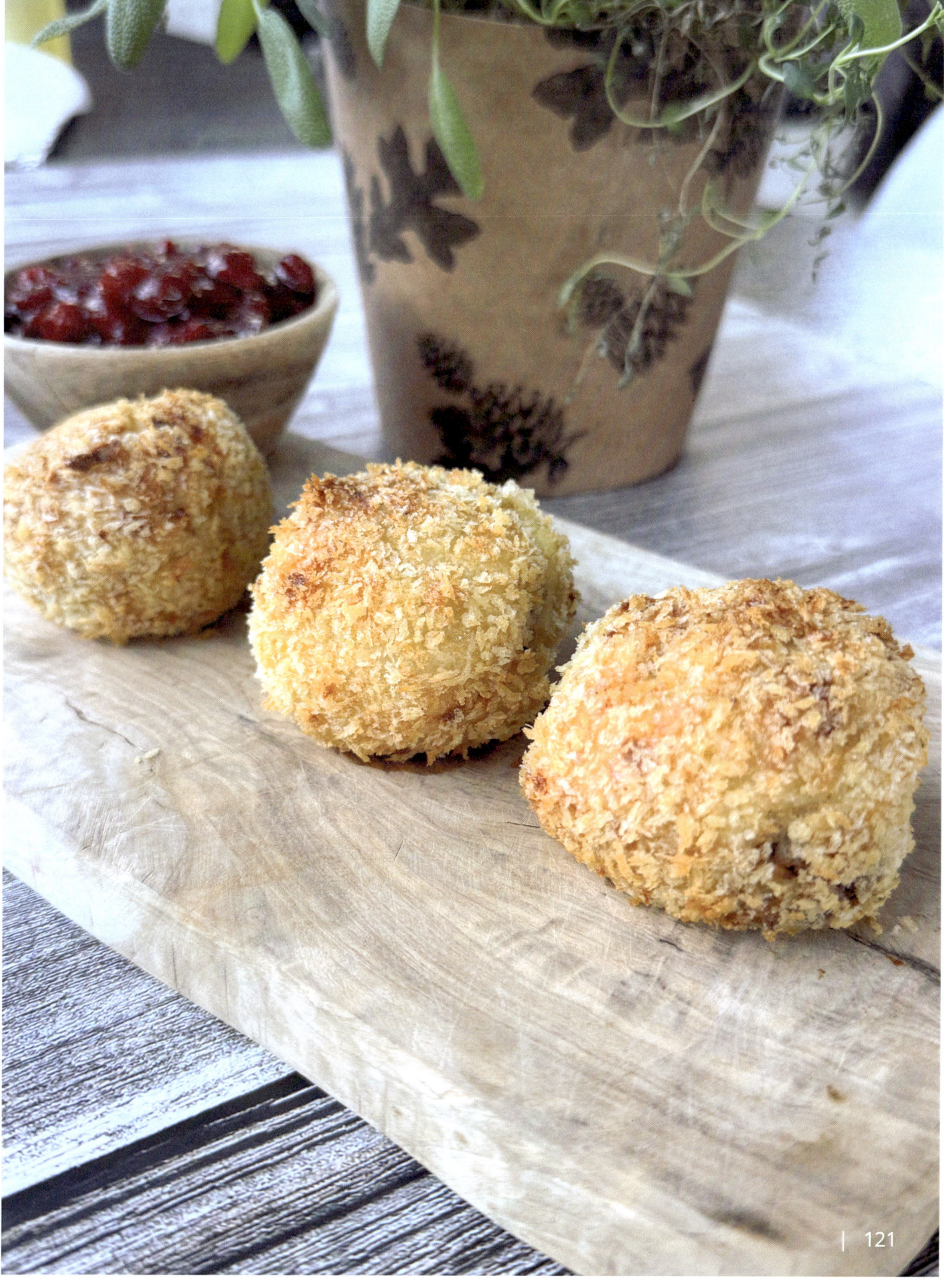

SWEET POTATO TURKEY SANDWICH

Sweet potatoes: not just a sad side dish anymore. Here, they star in a vibrant, low-carb, antioxidant-packed sandwich inspired by Okinawan longevity legends. We're layering purple sweet potatoes, turkey, and melty cheese for a mashup that's healthy and satisfying.

Ingredients

- **5 medium sweet potatoes, thinly sliced**
- **2 cups shredded cheese, mozzarella + Mexican blend**
- **1 tbsp oil**
- **Salt & pepper to taste**
- **8 slices turkey**
- **10 slices cheese, your favorite kind**
- **8 tomato slices**
- **Some lettuce or salad greens**
- **2 tbsp yellow mustard**
- **2 tbsp cranberry sauce or jam**
- **Sriracha to taste**
- **Cream cheese, optional for an extra creamy layer**

Instructions

- Preheat air fryer to 380°F. Line a 15x12-inch tray with parchment. Scatter an even layer of shredded cheese across the tray. Top with a single layer of sweet potato slices. Drizzle with oil and season lightly. Repeat layers: cheese, sweet potato, and a final cheese layer on top.
- Cook for 20 minutes, until the potatoes are tender and cheese is golden.
- Drizzle mustard over one half of the cooked sweet potato sheet. Layer with sliced cheese, turkey, more cheese. Fold the other half of the sheet over.
- Return to the air fryer or oven for 5–10 minutes, until everything inside is melted.
- Open each sandwich slice and stuff with tomato, lettuce and cranberry sauce.

Scan to watch

Serves 4

Prep time
10 min

Cook time
30 min

Quick Tips:
- Mandolin = your BFF: Thin, even slices make the sandwich layers cook evenly and stay sturdy.
- Swap turkey for ham, try smoked gouda instead of Mexican blend.
- Don't skip the cranberry sauce + sriracha—it's the flavor bomb.

Calories: ~320 | Protein: ~25g | Carbs: ~18g | Fat: ~16g

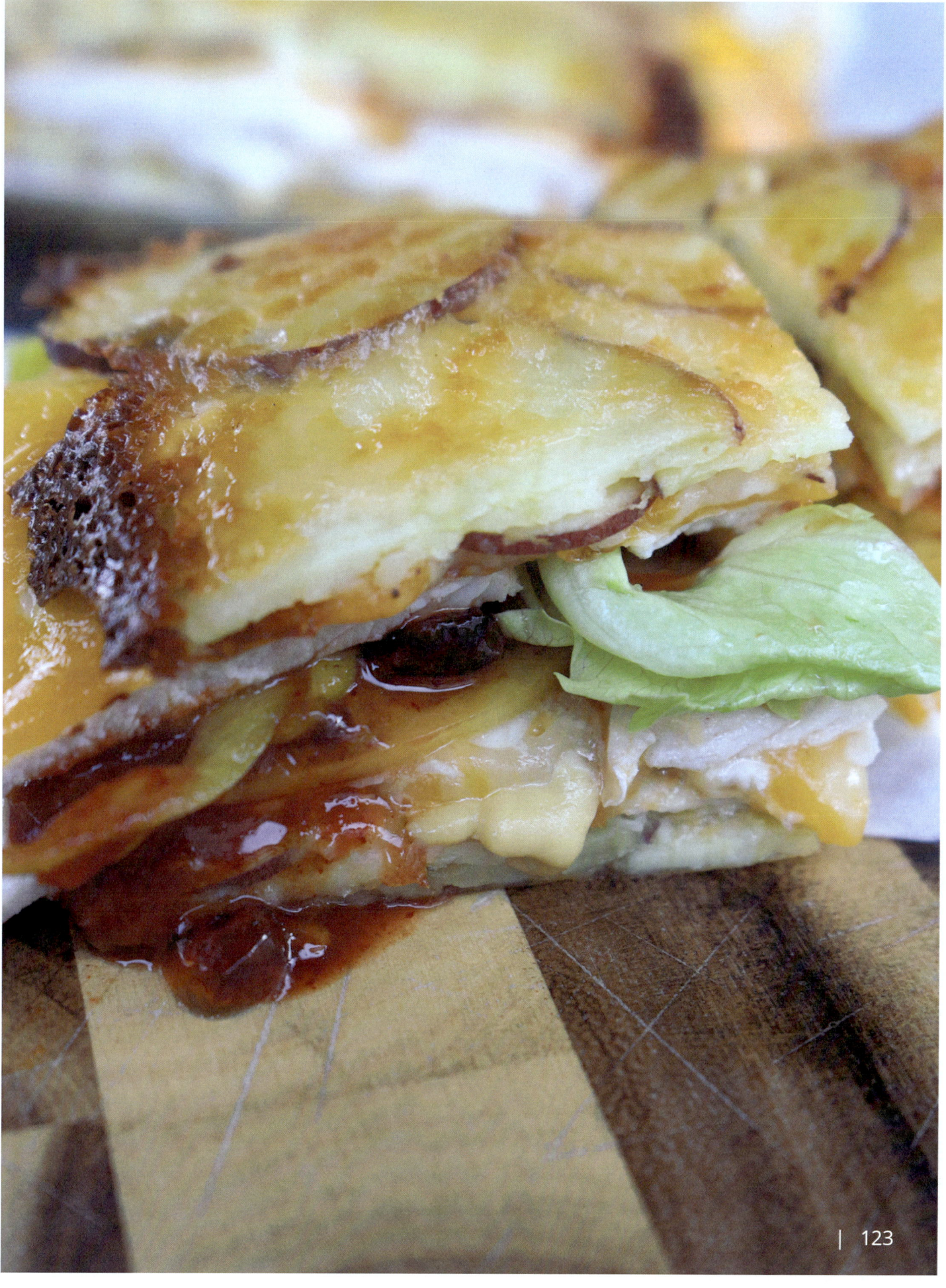

LEMON HERB WHOLE FISH

This is not your average "fish and potatoes" dinner. This is rustic, elegant, no-fuss cooking that looks—and smells—like Mediterranean vacation.. Bonus: it's packed with protein, low in carbs, and requires only one sheet pan.

Ingredients

For the Fish:
- **1 whole fish (sea bass, snapper), cleaned and scaled**
- **Optional: fillets of barramundi**
- **2 tbsp garlic spread**
- **2 tbsp olive oil**
- **1 tsp paprika**
- **1 tsp Italian seasoning**
- **Salt and pepper to taste**
- **1 lemon, sliced into rounds**
- **Fresh dill and parsley for garnish**

For the Potato Sidekick:
- **5 potatoes, thinly sliced**
- **2 tbsp olive oil**
- **1 tbsp fruit vinegar (apple cider or white balsamic)**
- **1 tsp paprika**
- **Salt and pepper, to taste**
- **1 onion, thinly sliced**
- **1 cup cherry tomatoes**

Instructions

- Preheat your oven to 400°F.
- In a small bowl, stir together garlic spread, olive oil, paprika, Italian seasoning, salt, and pepper. Stuff a few lemon slices, parsley, and dill inside.
- Toss the thin potato slices with olive oil, vinegar, paprika, salt, and pepper. Spread them across the tray. Top with thinly sliced onion and scatter cherry tomatoes.
- Place the seasoned fish right on top of the potato bed, If you're using barramundi fillets too, snuggle them around the potatoes.
- Slide the tray into the oven and bake for 25–30 minutes, until the fish flakes easily and the potatoes are golden and slightly crispy at the edges.

Scan to watch

Serves 4

Prep time
15 min

Cook time
30 min

Quick Tips:
- Grab fillets and reduce bake time to about 15 minutes.
- Crispier potatoes: spread them out in a single, even layer.

Calories: ~320 | Protein: ~25g | Carbs: ~18g | Fat: ~15g

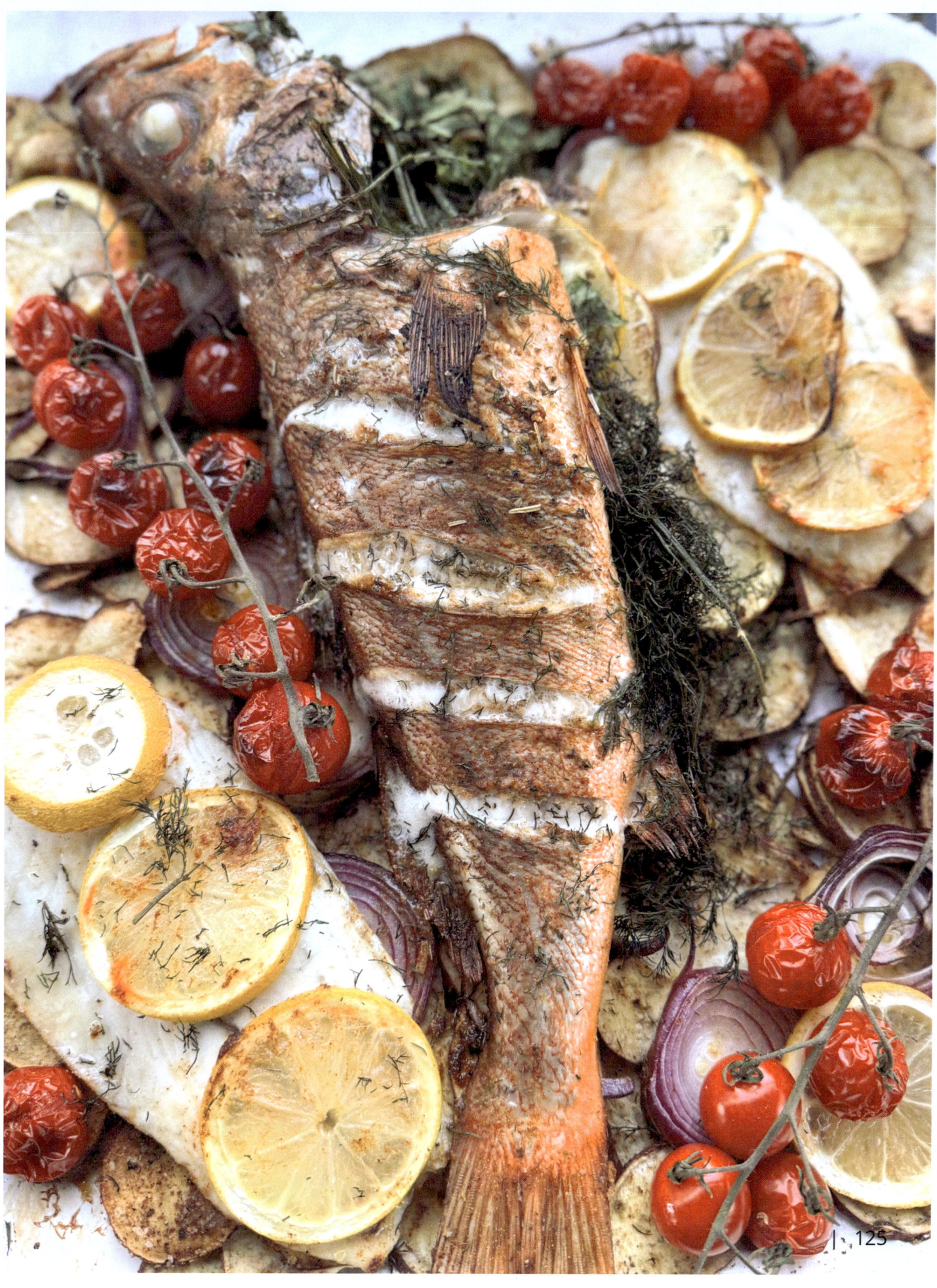

INSTANT POT MEXICAN BIRRIA TACOS

If comfort food wore a crown, birria tacos would be it. These tacos are smoky, cheesy, saucy, and ridiculously satisfying. And thanks to the Instant Pot, you don't have to slow cook for hours—unless that's your thing.

Ingredients

For the Meat & Sauce:
- 3 lbs chuck roast, 2" slices
- Salt and pepper, to taste
- Oil for searing
- 4–5 guajillo peppers
- 2–3 ancho peppers
- 1–2 chipotle peppers
- 2–3 pasilla peppers
- 2 medium tomatoes
- 1 onion, roughly chopped
- 5 garlic cloves

Seasonings:
- 1 tsp ground cumin
- 1 tsp dried oregano
- 1 tsp ground coriander
- 1 tsp paprika
- Pinch of ground cloves
- 2 bay leaves
- 1 cinnamon stick
- Salt & pepper to taste
- 2 cups beef broth

For the Tacos:
- 20 tortillas (corn or flour)

Instructions

- Set your Instant Pot to sauté mode. Sear beef cubes in batches until browned. Remove and set aside.
- Soak dried peppers in hot water for 10 minutes. Then blend with tomatoes, onion, and garlic until smooth.
- Pour sauce into the Instant Pot. Add all the seasonings, bay leaves, cinnamon stick, and seared beef. Pour in beef broth. Seal it and cook on high for 60 minutes. Natural release for 15 min.
- Shred the beef with two forks. Dip tortillas in the sauce.
- In a hot skillet, add dipped tortilla, sprinkle cheese, and load with shredded beef. Fold and crisp both sides until golden brown.
- Garnish with cilantro, onion, radish, and a good squeeze of lime.

Scan to watch

20 Tacos

Prep time
20 min

Cook time
1h, 15min

Quick Tips:
- Bonus: the leftover sauce makes the BEST birria soup. Add beans, chicken, or leftover beef and simmer for 10–15 min.
- No Instant Pot? Use a Dutch oven and slow cook for 3–4 hours.

(Per Taco): 200 calories | 15g protein | 10g carbs | 10g fat

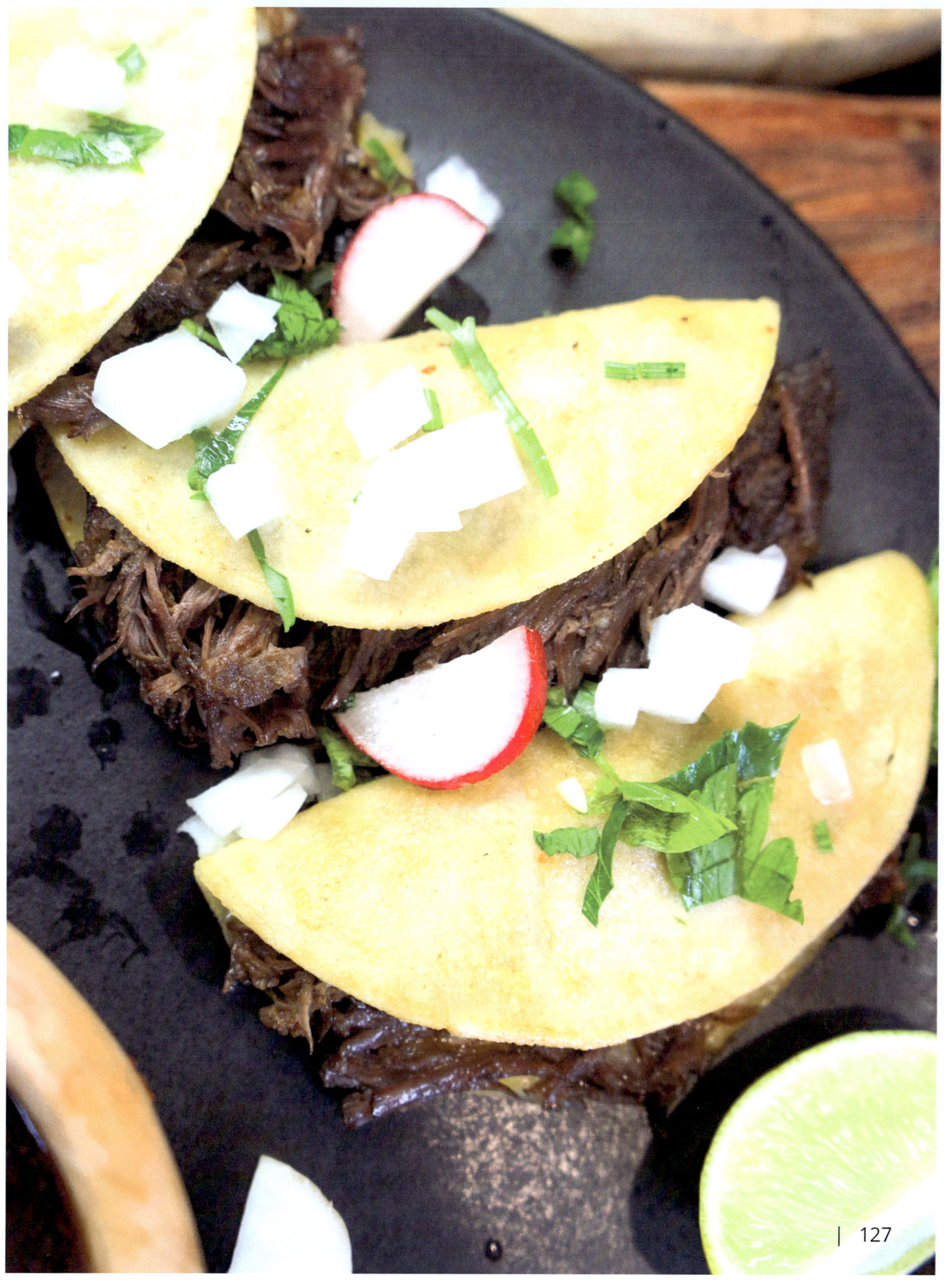

THAI-INSPIRED CHICKEN MEATBALLS

This is what happens when meatballs go on vacation to Thailand. Inspired by a fish curry I whipped up not long ago, this dish is fast, bold, and high-protein enough to impress your muscles and your taste buds.

Ingredients

For the Chicken Meatballs:
- 2 lbs ground chicken
- 1 stalk lemongrass
- ginger 3-inch, grated
- 3 garlic cloves
- 1 red chili, roughly chopped
- Handful of fresh cilantro
- 1 tbsp coconut aminos
- 1 tsp fish sauce
- 3 tbsp sesame oil (for frying)

For the Coconut Curry Sauce:
- 2 tbsp vegetable oil
- 1 onion, finely chopped
- 3 garlic cloves, minced
- ginger 1-inch, grated
- 2 stalks lemongrass
- 2 Thai red chilies
- 2 tsp turmeric powder
- 2 tsp ground coriander
- 1 tbsp red curry paste
- 2 (14 oz) cans coconut milk
- 1 tbsp fish sauce
- Zest + juice of 1 lime

Instructions

- Blend lemongrass, ginger, garlic, chili, cilantro, coconut aminos, fish sauce, and collagen (if using). Mix into ground chicken and roll into 18 meatballs.
- Heat sesame oil in a skillet, brown meatballs on all sides. Set aside.
- In the same pan, sauté onion, garlic, and ginger in oil. Add bruised lemongrass, chilies, turmeric, coriander, curry paste, and lime zest. Stir until fragrant.
- Pour in coconut milk, lime juice, and fish sauce. Simmer 10 min. Add meatballs and cook 5 min more.
- Combine jasmine rice, coconut milk, water, and a pinch of salt in a pot. Bring to a boil and simmer until the liquid is absorbed (about 15 minutes).
- Spoon rice into bowls, top with meatballs and sauce, garnish with cilantro.

Scan to watch

18 Meatballs

Prep time 15 min

Cook time 25 min

Quick Tips:
- Low-carb swap: ditch the rice and go with steamed veggies or cauliflower rice

Calories (3 meatballs): 450 | Protein: 38g | Carbs: 18g | Fat: 28g

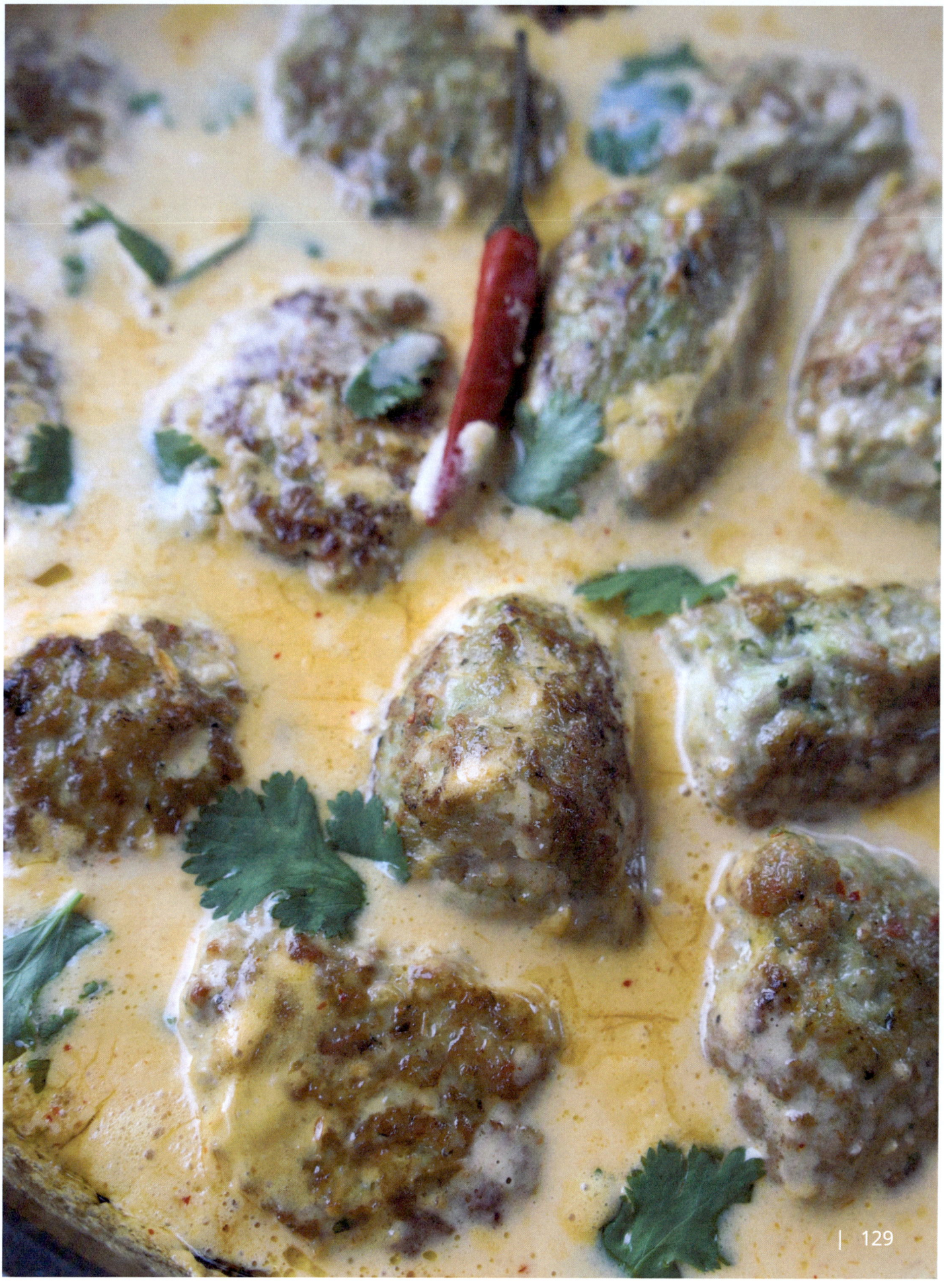

MEDITERRANEAN LAVASH ROLLS

Fresh, high-protein, and ready to roll—literally. These lavash wraps are loaded with creamy hummus, crisp veggies, and juicy shredded chicken. Great hot or cold, for lunch or a flex-worthy potluck dish.

Ingredients

Lavash Rolls:
- 3–4 lavash wraps
- ½ cup white bean hummus
- 1½ cups shredded chicken
- ½ cucumber, thinly sliced
- ½ bell pepper, thinly sliced
- ½ carrot, shredded
- Fresh parsley or cilantro

White Bean Hummus:
- 1 can (15 oz) white beans
- 2 tbsp tahini
- 1 tbsp olive oil
- 1 garlic clove
- Juice of 1 lemon
- ½ tsp cumin
- Salt to taste
- Water, as needed

Shredded Chicken:
- 3 frozen chicken thighs
- 1 cup chicken broth
- 1 tsp each: garlic powder, onion powder, paprika
- Salt & pepper
- Lemon juice, olives

Instructions

- Make the hummus: blend all ingredients until smooth. Add water as needed.
- Cook the chicken: add chicken, broth, and seasonings to Instant Pot. Pressure cook for 15 min, natural release for 5. Shred and mix with lemon juice, olives if using.
- Assemble rolls: spread hummus on lavash. Add chicken, veggies, and herbs. Roll tightly, fold ends, slice.

Scan to watch

3 rolls

Prep time 15 min

Cook time 15 min

Quick Tips:
- Want sauce? Mix Greek yogurt, tahini, lemon, and garlic powder.
- Use frozen chicken straight in the Instant Pot.
- Store components separately; assemble when eating.
- No tahini? No problem. Swap it with natural peanut butter for a creamy, nutty twist on the hummus.

Calories (per roll): ~280 | Protein: ~20g | Carbs: ~25g | Fat: ~10g

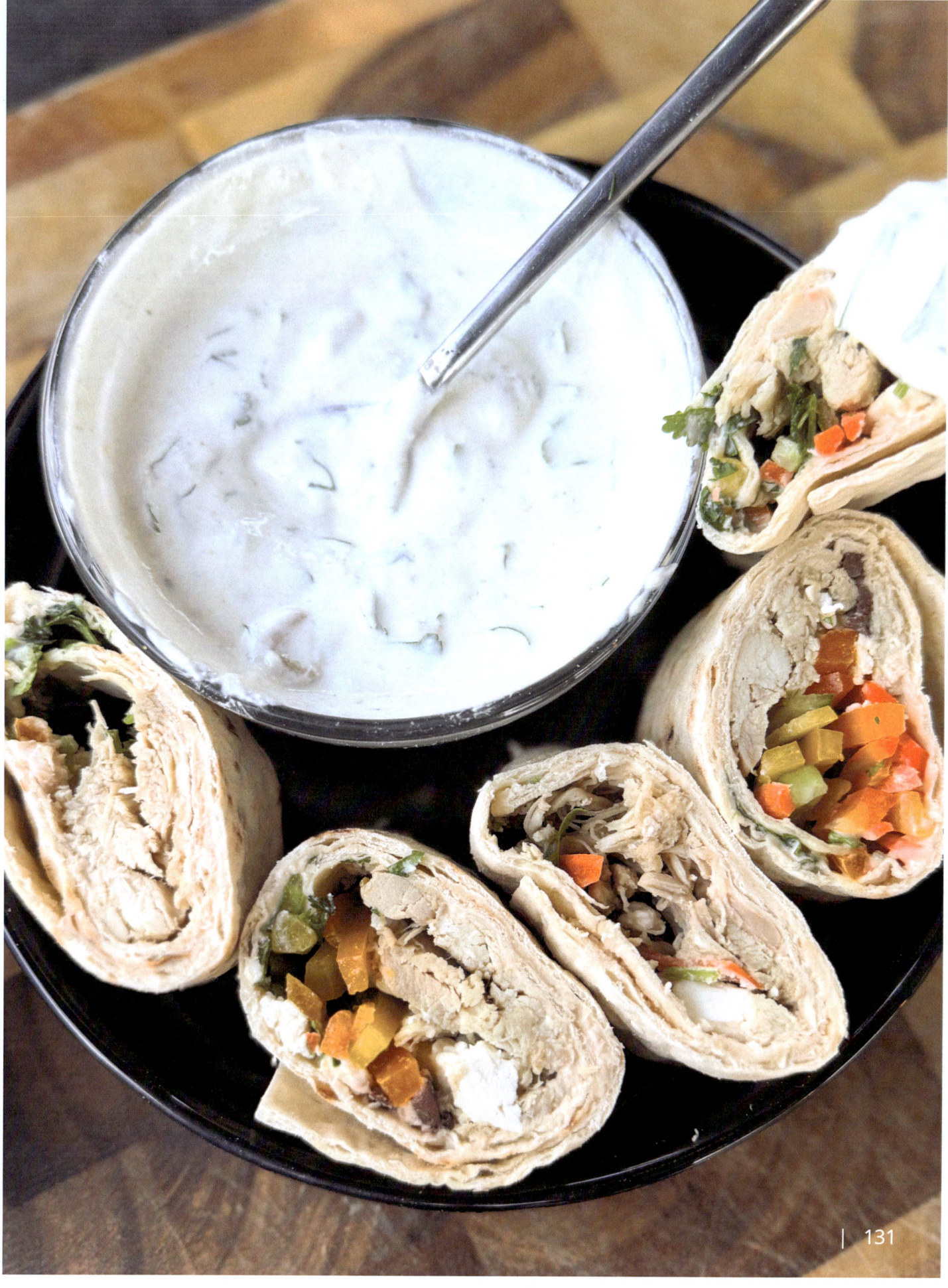

CHICKEN PASTA PUTTANESCA

Puttanesca is all about bold, briny flavors and getting things done with minimal effort. We've amped it up with crispy chicken legs and high-protein pasta to make it a filling, flavorful meal.

Ingredients

- **Oil for frying**
- **6 chicken legs (bone-in, skin-on)**
- **Salt & pepper**
- **Juice of 1 lemon**
- **4 anchovy fillets, chopped**
- **2 tbsp capers, drained**
- **½ cup Kalamata olives, halved**
- **4 garlic cloves, minced**
- **1 can (28 oz) San Marzano tomatoes**
- **1 tsp red pepper flakes**
- **1 tsp dried oregano**
- **1 tsp Italian seasoning**
- **12 oz pasta (whole-grain or high-protein)**
- **½ cup reserved pasta water**
- **¼ cup fresh parsley**
- **¼ cup Parmesan, for serving**

Instructions

- Boil pasta in salted water until al dente. Reserve ½ cup water, drain, and set aside.
- Heat oil in a large skillet. Season chicken with salt, pepper, and lemon juice. Fry ~8–10 mins per side until golden and cooked through. Set aside.
- In the same skillet, add anchovies and stir until melted. Add garlic, capers, olives, red pepper flakes, oregano, and Italian seasoning. Sauté 2 mins. Pour in tomatoes and break them up. Simmer 10 mins.
- Toss cooked pasta into the sauce. Add pasta water as needed. Nestle chicken legs into skillet. Spoon sauce on top and heat through for 2–3 mins.
- Plate pasta and top with chicken, Parmesan, and parsley.

Scan to watch

Serves 4

Prep time 10 min

Cook time 20 min

Quick Tips:
- Anchovy melt into umami flavor—don't skip.
- Bone-in chicken = flavor bomb. Boneless works too for faster prep.
- Too thick? Add pasta water, not more oil.
- Batch it: Sauce freezes great without the pasta.

Calories: ~420 | Protein: ~35g | Carbs: ~35g | Fat: ~18g

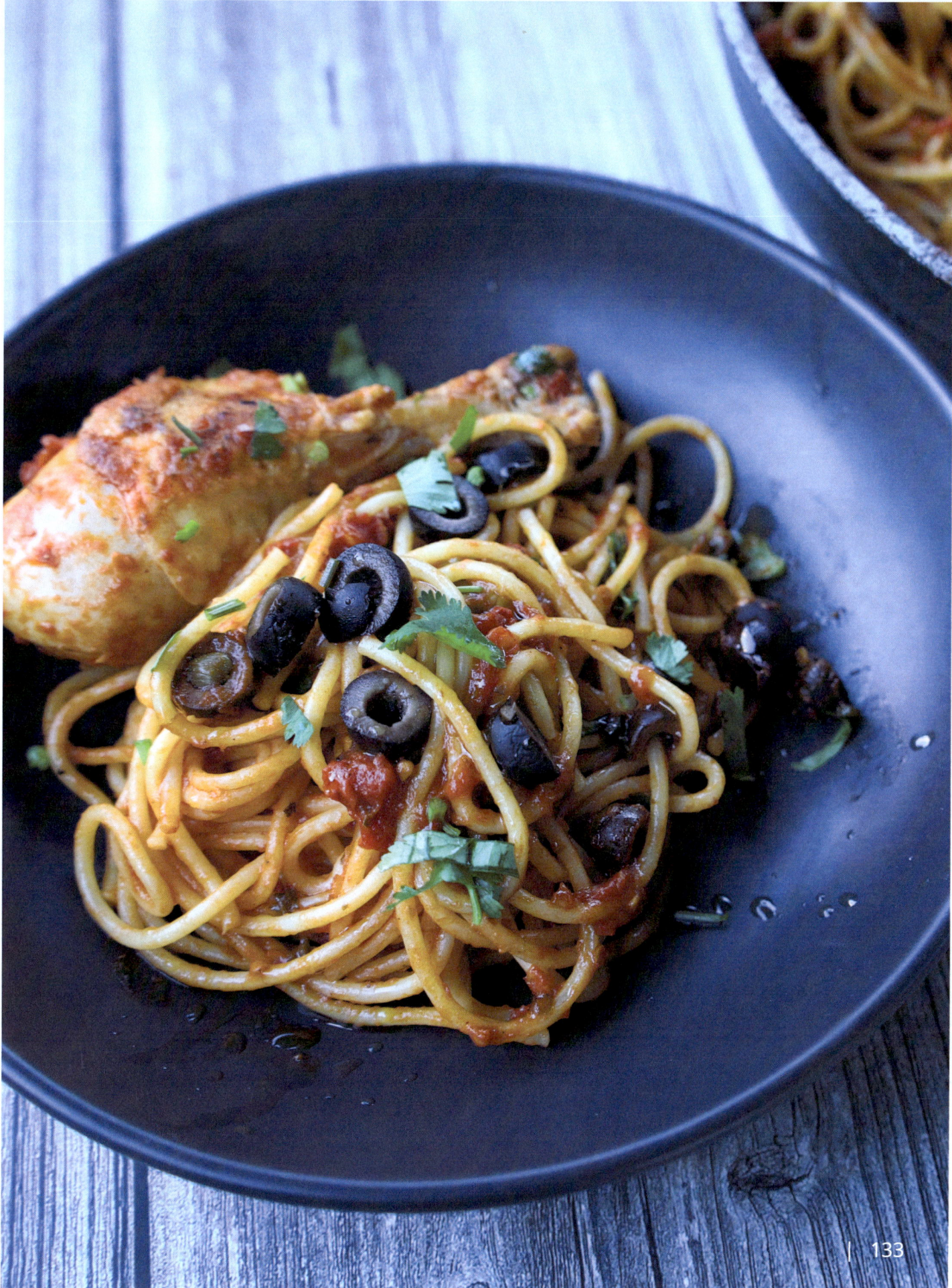

ONE-POT PERI PERI CHICKEN & RICE BAKE

This is your one-pot wonder when you want big flavor and even bigger protein—with very little mess. Think spicy chicken meets cozy rice pilaf. Bonus: it's all baked together, and you barely have to think.

Ingredients

For the Chicken:
- 4–6 bone-in, chicken thighs
- ½ cup peri peri sauce (store-bought or homemade)
- 2 tbsp olive oil
- 1 tsp smoked paprika
- ½ tsp garlic powder
- ½ tsp salt
- Juice of 1 lemon

For the Rice:
- 1½ cups basmati rice
- 2 cups chicken broth
- ¼ cup peri peri sauce
- 1 medium onion, diced
- 1 red bell pepper, diced
- 1 tsp smoked paprika
- ½ tsp ground cumin
- Salt and pepper, to taste

For Serving:
- Fresh cilantro
- Lime wedges
- Extra peri peri sauce

Instructions

- Toss chicken with peri peri sauce, olive oil, paprika, garlic powder, salt, and lemon juice. Marinate for at least 30 mins (or overnight).
- Preheat oven to 375°F. In a large casserole dish, mix rice, broth, peri peri sauce, onion, bell pepper, paprika, cumin, salt, and pepper.
- Place chicken on top (don't bury it). Cover tightly with foil and bake for 30 mins.
- Remove foil and bake another 10–15 mins until chicken is golden and rice is cooked.
- Let rest 5 mins. Top with cilantro, lime wedges, and extra peri peri sauce.

Scan to watch

Serves 6

Prep time
15 min

Cook time
45 min

Quick Tips:
- Want extra crispy skin? Broil the chicken for the last 2–3 minutes.
- This also works with boneless chicken, but the skin-on, bone-in thighs add major flavor.

Calories: 390 | Protein: 26g | Carbs: 32g | Fat: 15g

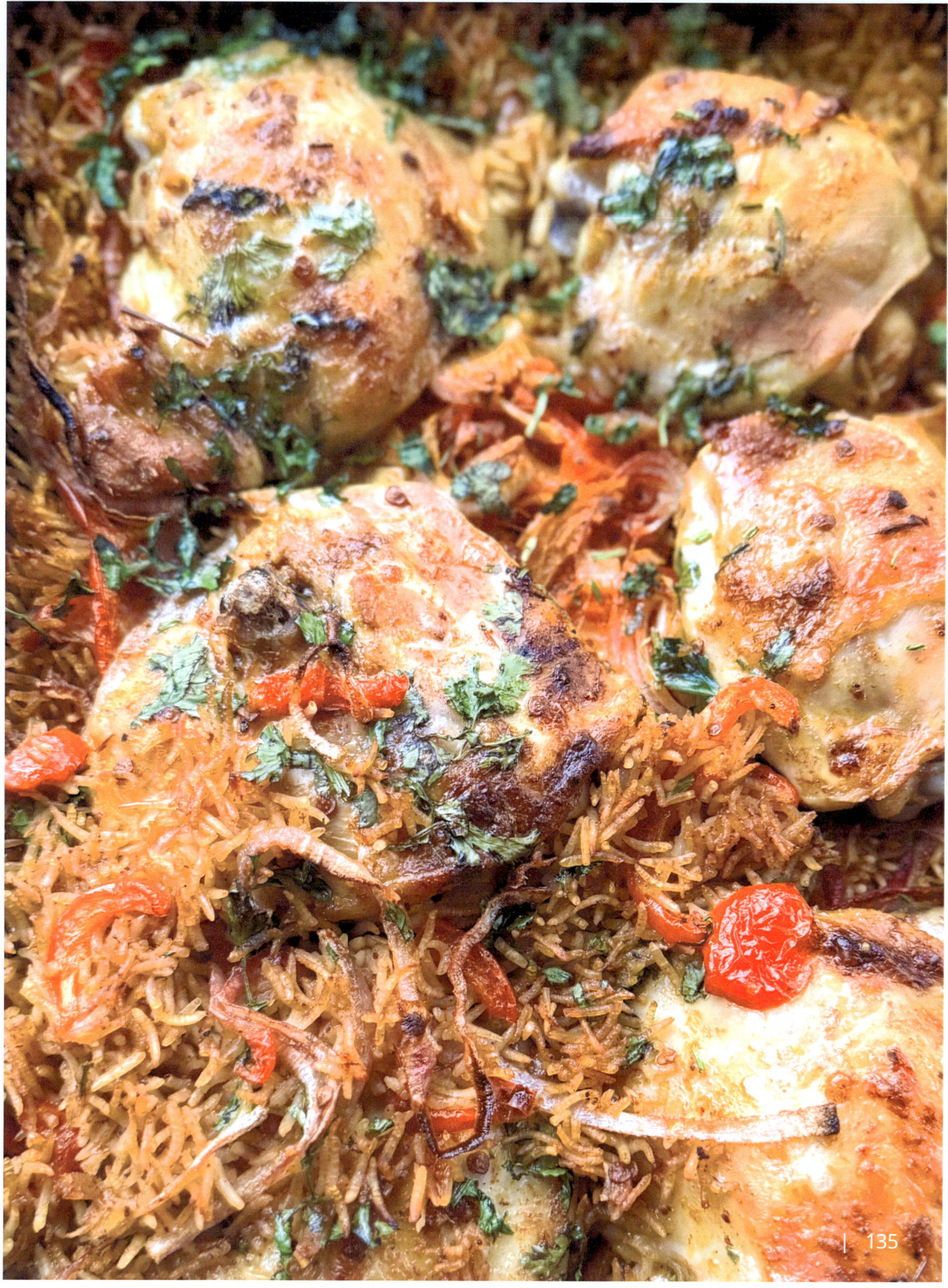

INSTANT POT PASTA BOLOGNESE

There's nothing quite like a comforting bowl of pasta Bolognese—especially one that doesn't demand hours of simmering. Inspired by a trip to Italy and supercharged for protein, this version leans on bacon, beef, and sausage for deep, rich flavor.

Ingredients

Meat & Veggies:
- 1 ½ cups chopped bacon
- 2 carrots, chopped
- 1 onion, chopped
- 5 garlic cloves, minced
- 2 lb ground beef
- 1 ½ cups cooked Italian sausage, chopped

Sauce Base:
- 1 ½ cups red wine
- 3 tbsp tomato paste
- 1 (28 oz) can San Marzano tomatoes
- 1 (14 oz) can tomato sauce
- 1 cup beef broth

Seasoning:
- Salt and pepper to taste
- 1 tsp Italian seasoning
- ½ tsp paprika

Pasta & Toppings:
- Pappardelle pasta, cooked separately
- Grated Parmesan

Instructions

- Set Instant Pot to sauté. Cook chopped bacon until crispy. Remove and set aside.
- In the same pot, sauté carrots, onion, and garlic until soft. Add ground beef and cook until browned.
- Stir in wine, tomato paste, San Marzano tomatoes, tomato sauce, and broth. Add Italian sausage, seasonings, and return bacon to the pot. Mix well.
- Seal the lid and pressure cook on high for 20 minutes. Let the pressure release naturally for 10 minutes.
- While the sauce cooks, boil pappardelle in salted water until al dente. Reserve some pasta water.
- Mix pasta with the Bolognese sauce. Add a splash of pasta water if needed. Top with Parmesan and basil.

Scan to watch

Serves 8

Prep time
15 min

Cook time
35 min

Quick Tips:
- Batch it: freeze leftover sauce in silicone muffin molds for easy single servings later.
- Make it lighter: use ground turkey instead of beef and sausage for a leaner version.

Calories: 424 | Protein: 24g | Carbs: 30g | Fat: 21g

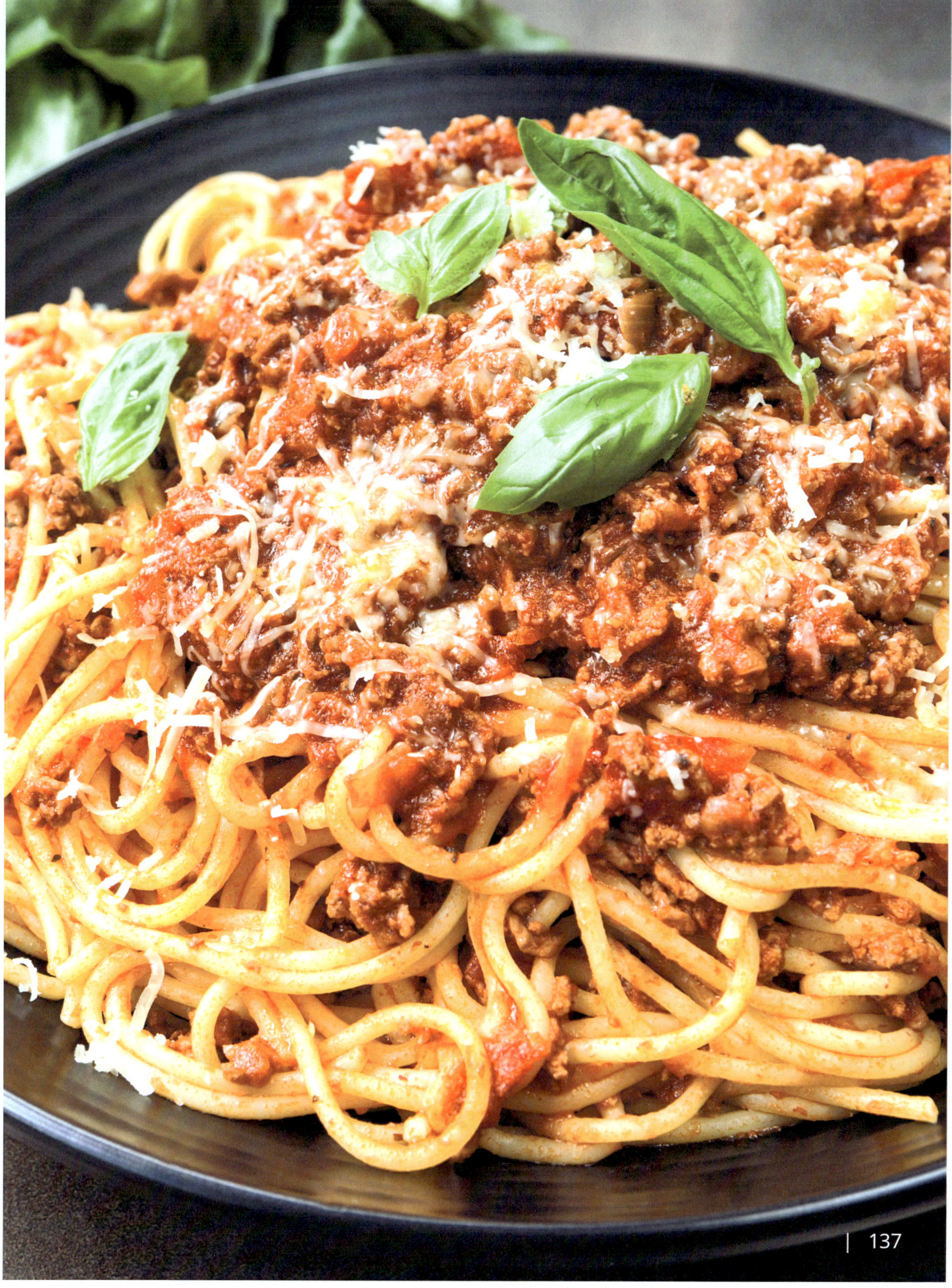

PORK CHOPS IN LEMON CAPER SAUCE

This dish hits every note—juicy pork chops, a zesty lemon caper sauce, creamy beans, and just enough tender cabbage to make you feel like a health-conscious adult. All done in 30 minutes.

Ingredients

- **4 bone-in pork chops (about 1 inch thick)**
- **2 tbsp olive oil**
- **3 garlic cloves, minced**
- **1 cup chicken stock**
- **1/3 cup fresh lemon juice (about 2 lemons)**
- **1 tbsp Dijon mustard**
- **2 tbsp capers, drained**
- **1 cup cooked cannellini or Great Northern beans (rinsed if canned)**
- **4 cups shredded cabbage**
- **Salt and freshly ground black pepper, to taste**
- **Fresh parsley, chopped (for garnish)**
- **Optional: roasted baby potatoes for serving**

Instructions

- Pat dry pork chops, then season generously with salt and pepper.
- Heat 1 tbsp olive oil in a large skillet over medium-high. Sear chops for 4 minutes per side until golden. Remove and set aside.
- In the same skillet, add 1 tbsp olive oil and cabbage. Sauté 2–3 minutes until softened. Remove and set aside.
- Sauté garlic for 30 seconds. Add chicken stock, lemon juice, Dijon mustard, and capers. Stir well. Toss in the beans and return the cabbage to the pan.
- Nestle pork chops back in. Spoon sauce and veggies over the top. Simmer 5–10 minutes until internal temp hits 145°F.
- Plate chops with cabbage-bean mix and spoon that lemony sauce all over.

Scan to watch

Serves 4

Prep time
10 min

Cook time
20 min

Quick Tips:
- Sear in batches: If your skillet isn't large enough, sear the pork chops in batches to avoid overcrowding.
- Add a splash of wine: A splash of dry white wine in the sauce takes it to restaurant-level flavor.

Calories: 380 | Protein: 40g | Carbs: 12g | Fat: 18g

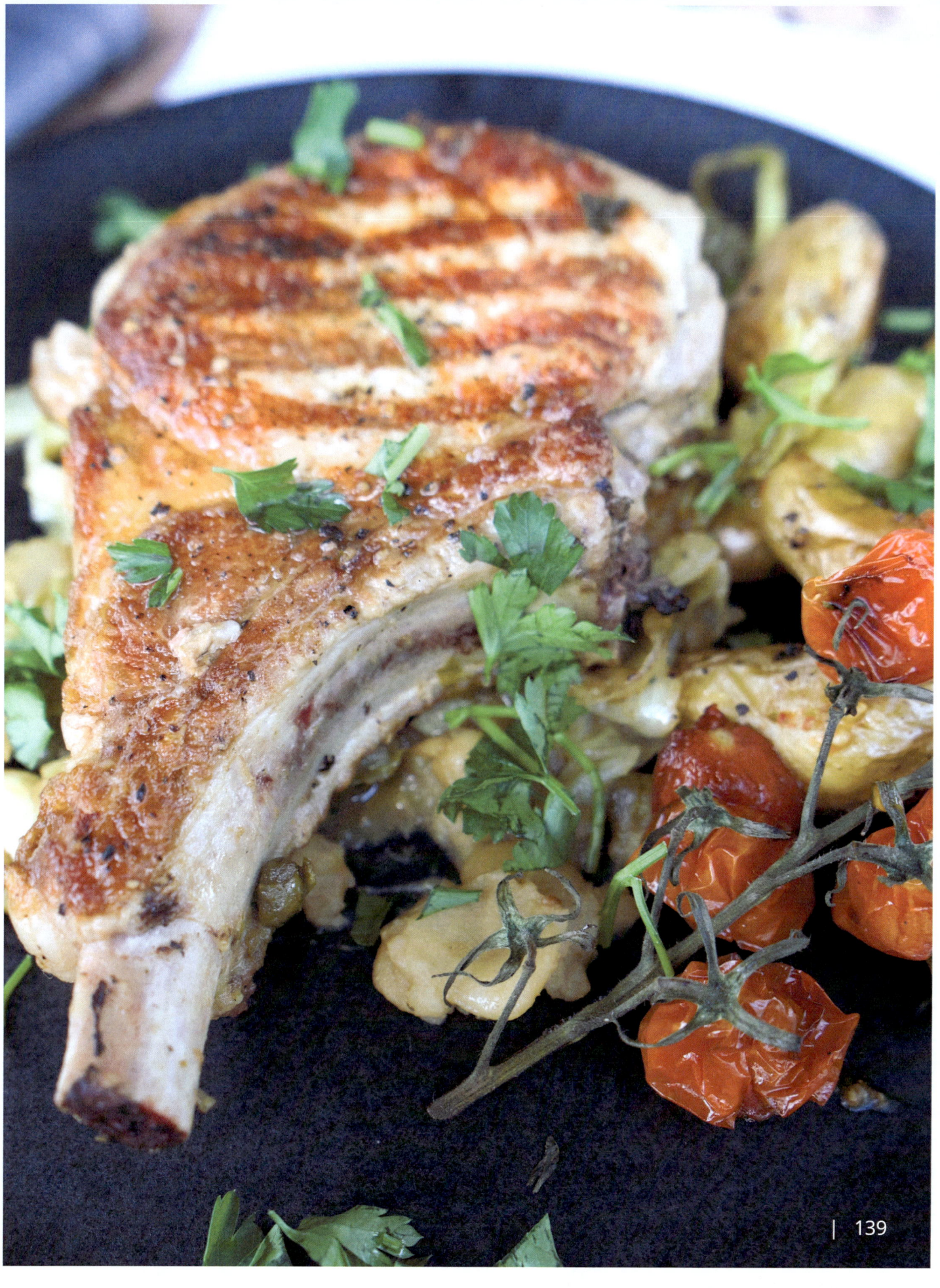

THREE TOMATOES CHICKEN & BEANS

If you love a hearty tomato sauce, this dish is for you. It's saucy, savory, and perfect for unwinding after a long day. Make it in the Instant Pot for a quick option, or stick to the skillet for that perfect sear.

Ingredients

- **7 chicken thighs**
- **Salt & pepper to taste**
- **4 strips bacon, chopped**
- **Oil for frying**
- **2 apples, sliced**
- **1 onion, chopped**
- **4 garlic cloves, minced**
- **2 tbsp tomato paste**
- **1 tsp red pepper flakes**
- **1 tsp paprika**
- **1 tsp thyme**
- **1 tsp oregano**
- **5 heirloom tomatoes, sliced**
- **1 can (14 oz) San Marzano tomatoes**
- **2 cans (14 oz each) cooked butter beans**
- **Fresh basil for garnish**

Instructions

- Heat a large skillet over medium-high heat with a drizzle of oil. Sear the chicken thighs until golden brown. Remove and set aside.
- Add the chopped bacon to the skillet. Cook until crispy, then remove and set aside.
- Add the sliced apples, onion, and garlic to the skillet. Sauté until the onion is translucent and the apples soften.
- Stir in the tomato paste and seasonings. Add the heirloom tomatoes, canned San Marzano tomatoes, and butter beans. Bring to a simmer.
- Nestle the chicken and bacon into the sauce. Cover and simmer for 25-30 minutes, stirring occasionally.
- Top with fresh basil and plate it up!

Scan to watch

Serves 7

Prep time 10 min

Cook time 35 min

Quick Tips:
- For a faster version, sauté the chicken, bacon, and veggies, then add everything else and cook on high for 10 minutes.
- If heirloom tomatoes aren't available, use regular tomatoes.

Calories: ~340 | Protein: ~28g | Carbs: ~24g | Fat: ~15g

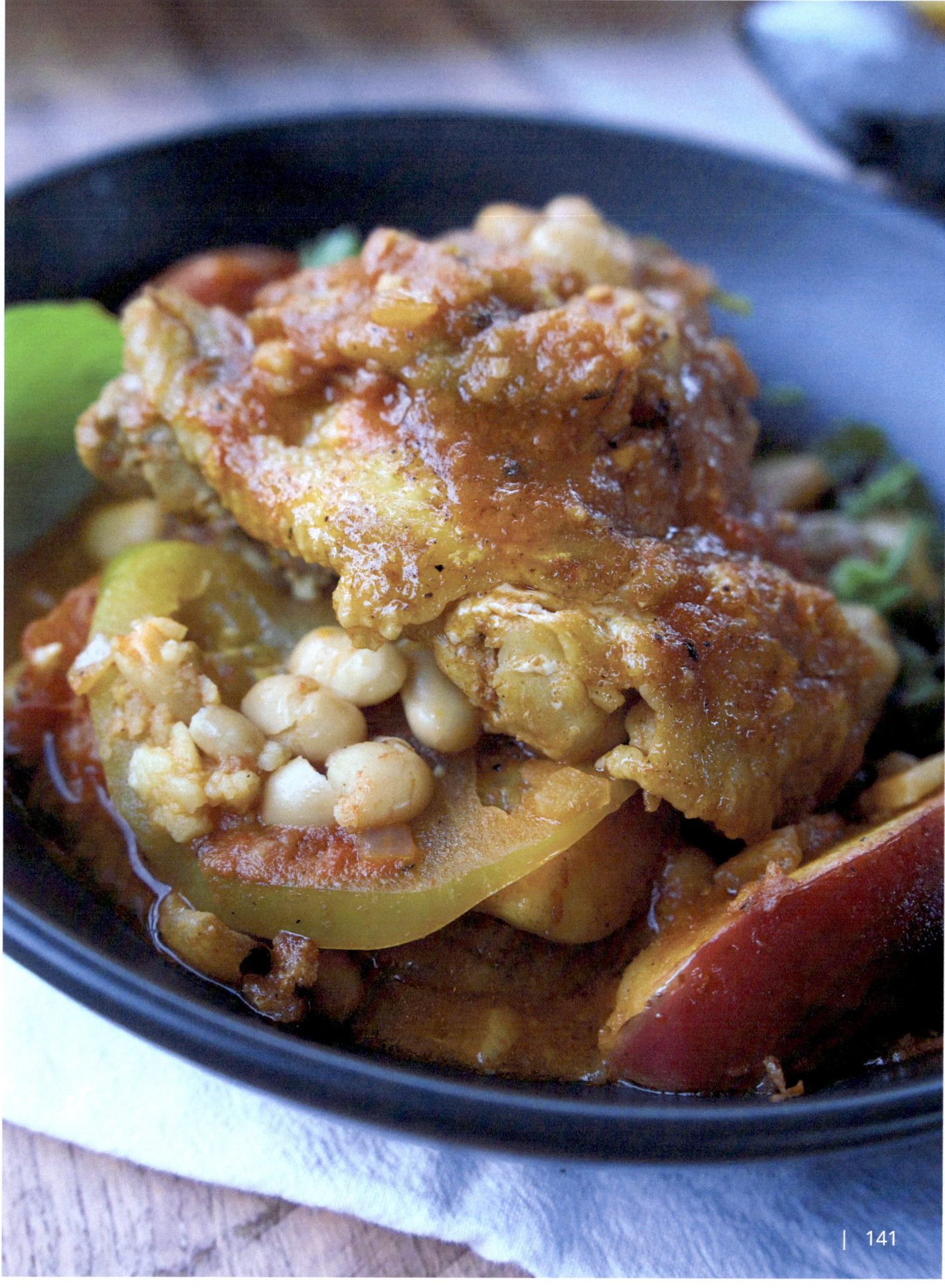

SALMON POWER BOWL

Almost a poke bowl—but cooked. This 30-minute protein-loaded meal is fast, flavorful, and surprisingly kid-approved. Great for lunch, dinner, or that weird in-between "I should've eaten an hour ago" moment.

Ingredients

Salmon:
- 1.5–2 lb salmon
- 2 tsp liquid smoke
- Juice of ½ lemon
- Salt and pepper to taste
- Dill to taste
- Sriracha seasoning to taste

Rice:
- 2 cups cooked brown rice (Instant Pot recommended)
- Furikake seasoning to taste

Toppings:
- Salad greens, corn, parsley, scallions, cucumbers, marinated ginger, wasabi, sesame seeds, edamame

Sauces:
- Sriracha mayo (mayo + sriracha + lime), ponzu, sweet chili sauce

Instructions

- Cook the salmon: preheat your air fryer to 390°F or heat a skillet over medium-high. Pat the salmon dry, then season with liquid smoke, lemon juice, salt, pepper, dill, and sriracha seasoning.
  - Air fryer method: Cook skin-side down for 10–12 minutes or until the salmon flakes easily with a fork.
- Prepare the rice: cook brown rice in the Instant Pot (use 1:1.25 rice-to-water ratio, pressure cook for 15 minutes, natural release). Mix in furikake while warm.
- Assemble bowls: start with a layer of rice, flake the cooked salmon on top, and pile on your chosen toppings.
- Sauce it up: drizzle with your preferred sauces right before serving.

Scan to watch

Serves 4

Prep time
10 min

Cook time
20 min

Quick Tips:
- Sub the brown rice for cauliflower rice or just double the greens.
- Cook extra salmon and rice to throw into wraps, salads, or scrambled eggs tomorrow.

Calories: ~520 | Protein: ~45g | Carbs: ~45g | Fat: ~18g

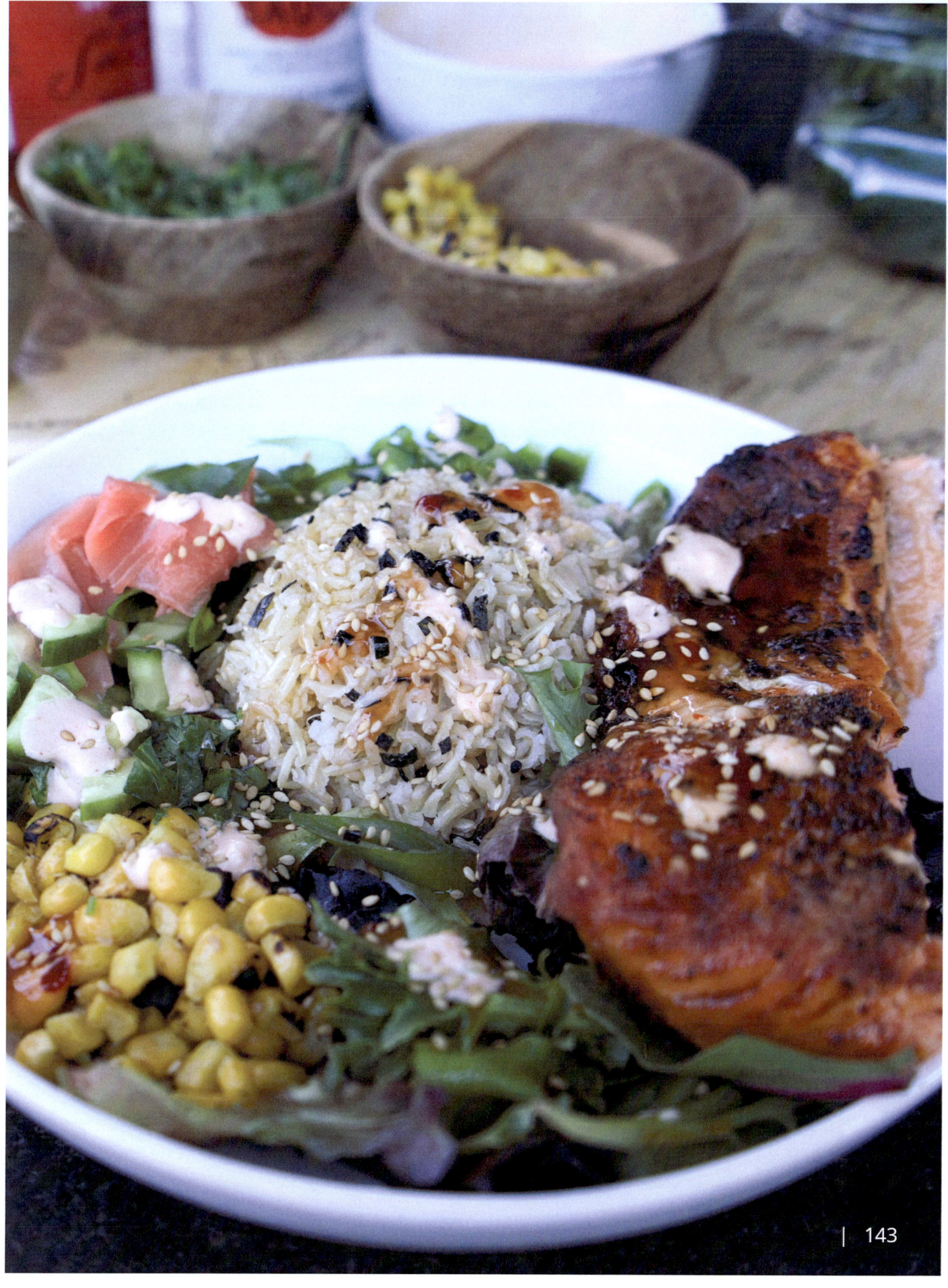

HIGH-PROTEIN POTATO GRATIN

You think potato gratin can't be gym-friendly? Think again. This protein-packed twist skips the cream, adds lean meat and beans, and sneaks in a whole lot of flavor. Perfect for meal prep or post-leg day refuel.

Ingredients

Base Layer:
- 1 shallot, chopped
- 2 bell peppers, chopped
- 4 garlic cloves, minced
- Oil, for sautéing
- 2 lb ground turkey
- Salt & pepper to taste
- 1 tsp each: paprika, cumin
- 2 cans (14 oz each) pinto beans, drained & rinsed

Cheesy Yogurt Sauce:
- 1 cup cottage cheese
- 1 cup Greek yogurt
- 1 tbsp Dijon mustard
- 2 sprigs fresh dill, chopped
- 2 cups Gruyère cheese, shredded (divided)
- Juice of 1 lemon
- ½ cup chicken broth

Potato Layers:
- 5–6 medium yellow or russet potatoes, thinly sliced
- Oil spray for baking dish

Instructions

- Preheat oven to 375°F. Spray baking dish with oil. Slice potatoes thin (use a mandolin if you've got one).
- Sauté shallot and bell peppers in a bit of oil (3–4 min), then add garlic. Stir in ground turkey and seasonings; cook until browned. Mix in beans and set aside.
- In a blender, combine cottage cheese, Greek yogurt, mustard, dill, lemon juice, and broth. Blend until smooth. Stir in 1 cup Gruyère.
- Layer half the potatoes, half the turkey mix, and half the sauce. Repeat. Top with remaining 1 cup Gruyère.
- Cover with foil and bake for 40 min, then uncover and bake 15–20 more until golden and bubbling.
- Let sit 10 min before slicing so it holds together.

Scan to watch

Serves 8

Prep time 20 min

Cook time 60 min

Quick Tips:
- Slice it into portions and freeze for easy post-workout meals.
- For the sauce: blend it warm (30 sec in microwave) for extra creaminess.

Calories: ~410 | Protein: ~38g | Carbs: ~35g | Fat: ~12g

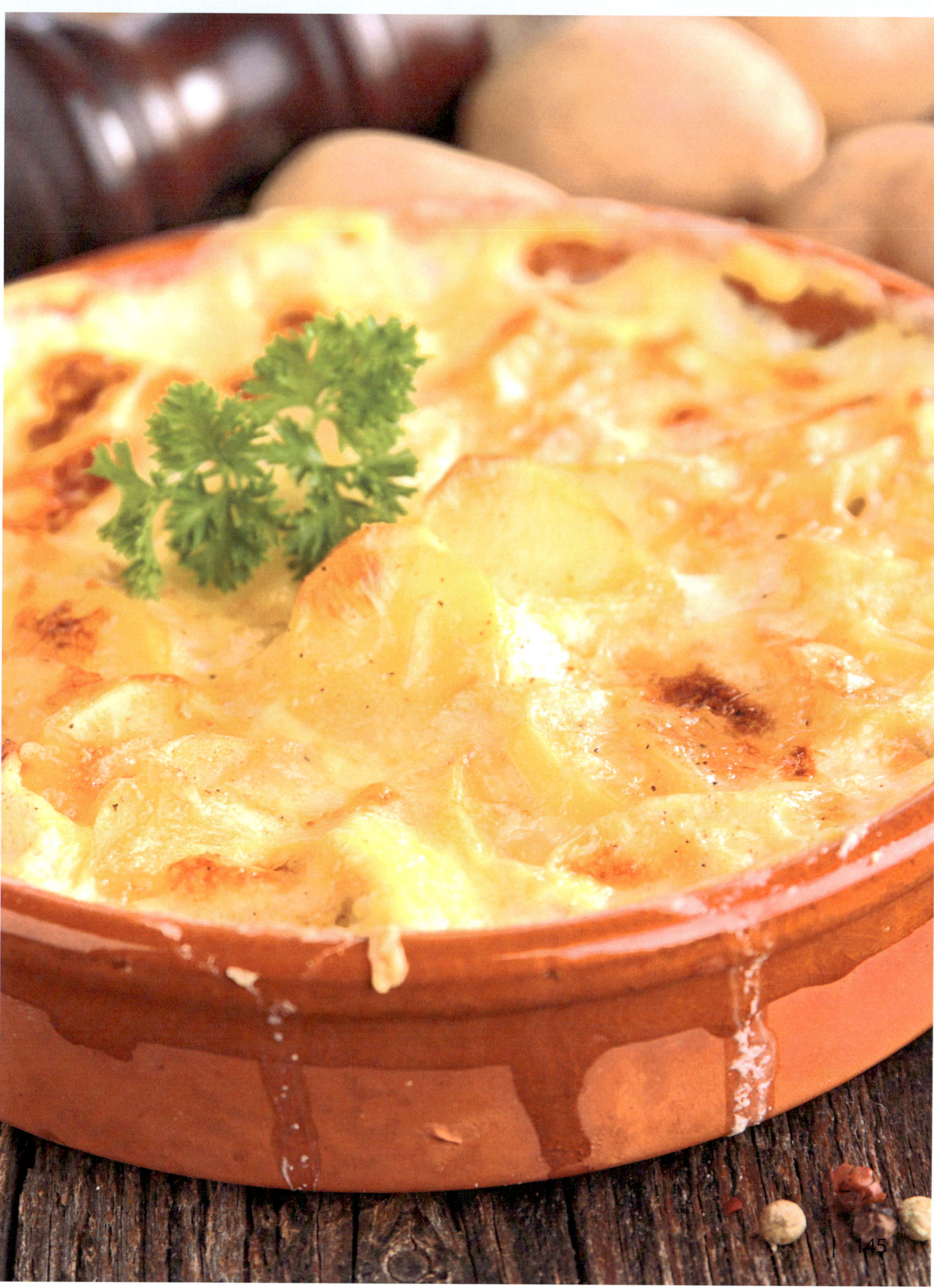

GOCHUJANG ROASTED WHOLE CHICKEN WITH CHARRED LEEKS & MISO-SPICED BEANS

Ever wonder how to get restaurant-quality flavor without the restaurant effort? This spicy-sweet roasted chicken packs heat and umami, and the miso-spiced beans with charred leeks make it a full, balanced plate.

Ingredients

For the Chicken:
- 1 whole chicken (~4–5 lbs)
- 3 tbsp gochujang
- 2 tbsp soy sauce
- 1 tbsp honey
- 1 tbsp rice vinegar
- 1 tbsp sesame oil
- 1½ tbsp orange juice
- 1 tsp garlic powder
- Salt & pepper to taste

For the Leeks & Miso Beans:
- 4 large leeks, chopped
- 1 tbsp sesame oil
- 1½ tbsp miso paste
- 4 cloves garlic, minced
- 1½ tbsp fresh ginger, minced
- Chili powder to taste
- 2 cans white beans
- 1 tbsp rice vinegar
- 1 tbsp soy sauce
- ½ cup chicken broth
- Thai basil & scallions

Instructions

- Marinate that bird: in a bowl, combine gochujang, soy sauce, honey, rice vinegar, sesame oil, orange juice, garlic powder, salt, and pepper. Rub it all over the chicken. Let it rest for 15–20 min.
- Roast it: preheat oven or air fryer to 425°F. Place chicken breast-side up in a roasting pan. Roast for 45–55 min, brushing with extra marinade in the last 5 minutes. Done when the thickest part hits 165°F.
- Make the leeks & beans: heat sesame oil in a large skillet. Sauté chopped leeks 5–7 minutes until browned and softened. Add garlic, ginger, miso, chili powder, rice vinegar, soy sauce, and broth. Stir, simmer 2 minutes. Add beans and stir to coat. Cook until heated through.

Scan to watch

Serves 6

Prep time 20 min

Cook time 55 min

Quick Tips:
- Time-saver: use pre-minced garlic and ginger to cut prep time.
- Fitness boost: want even more protein? Stir in some chopped cooked chicken breast to the bean mix for a post-workout meal.

Calories: ~420 | Protein: ~50g | Carbs: ~28g | Fat: ~12g

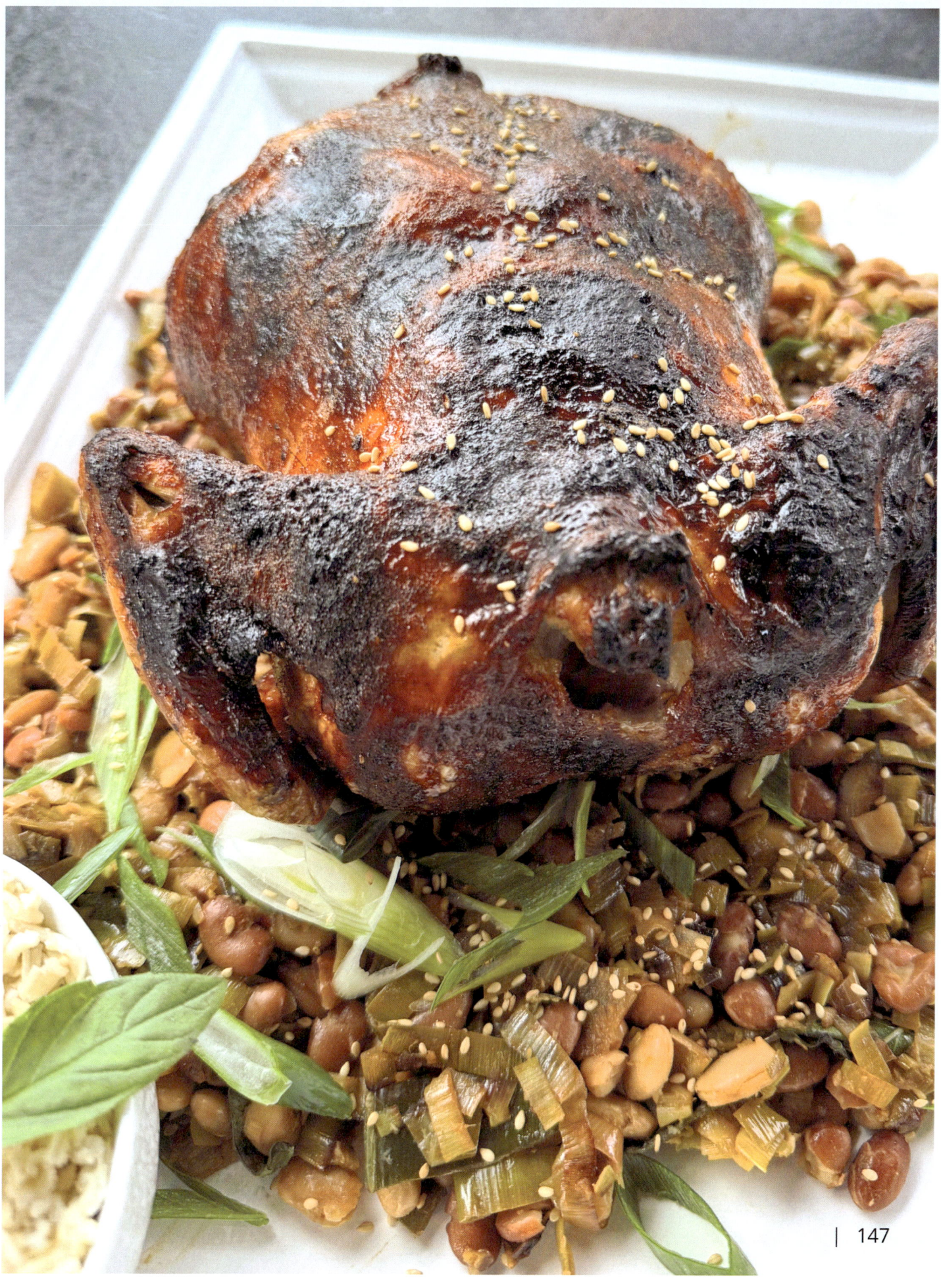

CHICKEN ON VEGGIE STACKS WITH MARINARA

I had friends coming over and zero time to make something elaborate. I threw together whatever was in the fridge—some drumsticks, leftover veggies, and made a quick marinara with fresh tomatoes. What came out of the oven looked like I'd planned it for days.

Ingredients

For the Chicken & Stacks:
- 8 chicken drumsticks (make 3 slits in each to soak up flavor)
- Salt & pepper to taste
- 3 toothpicks per drumstick
- 1 eggplant, thinly sliced
- 1 bell pepper, thinly sliced
- 1 onion, thinly sliced
- 2 potatoes, thinly sliced
- Mozzarella cheese, sliced

For the Marinara:
- 2 lbs fresh tomatoes, blended
- 1 onion, chopped
- 4 cloves garlic, minced
- Red pepper flakes to taste
- Oregano to taste
- Salt to taste
- 3 tbsp olive or avocado oil
- Fresh basil for garnish

Instructions

- Make the Marinara: blend tomatoes until smooth. Heat oil in a pan, sauté onions until soft, then add garlic, red pepper flakes, and oregano. Add tomatoes, simmer 15–20 min. Season with salt and stir in fresh basil.
- Season drumsticks with salt and pepper. Coat them in marinara and marinate for 30 minutes.
- Preheat oven to 400°F. Layer sliced eggplant, bell pepper, onion, potato, and mozzarella into small veggie towers. Top each with a marinated drumstick and secure with toothpicks.
- Transfer stacks to a baking dish. Spoon more marinara over and around the stacks. Cover with foil and bake for 45 minutes. Remove foil and bake 15 minutes more until the chicken is golden and cooked through.

Scan to watch

Serves 4

Prep time 25 min

Cook time 60 min

Quick Tips:
- Use a mandoline for thin, even veggie slices so the stacks stay tall and cook evenly. And don't skip the fresh basil.

Calories: ~380 | Protein: ~35g | Carbs: ~20g | Fat: ~15g

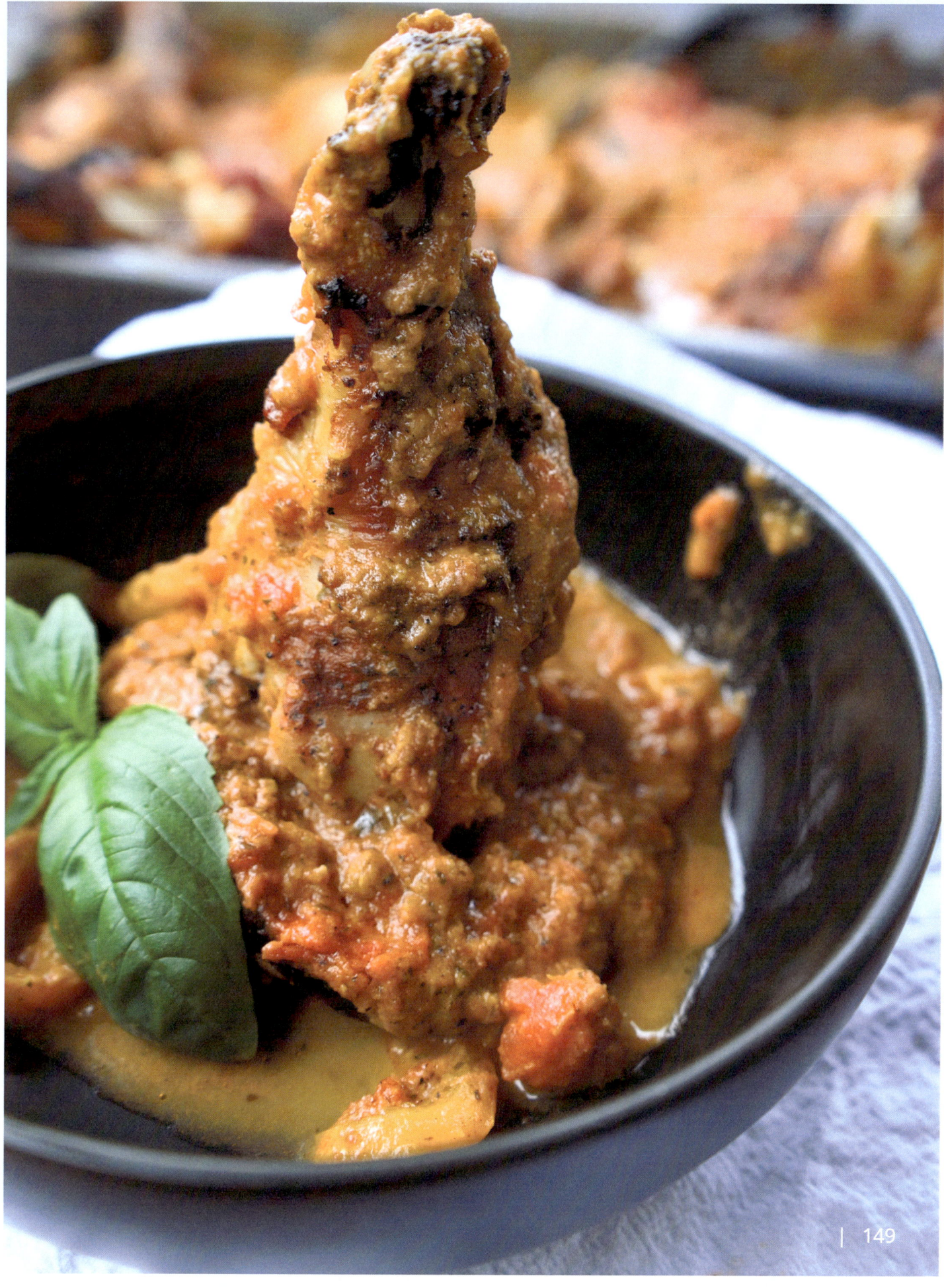

MOROCCAN CHICKEN MEAL PREP PIES

Let's be honest—meal prep can be soul-crushing. But not when you've got mini pies packed with warm Moroccan spices, crispy cauliflower crusts, and a zesty tabbouleh topper. These are satisfying and way more exciting than plain grilled chicken and broccoli.

Ingredients

Cauliflower Crust & Topping:
- 1 large head cauliflower, grated (or 2 ½ cups riced)
- 2 eggs
- 1 cup shredded Gruyère cheese
- 2 tbsp olive oil
- Salt & pepper to taste

Moroccan Chicken Filling:
- 2 boneless, skinless chicken breasts, cubed
- 1 tbsp olive oil
- 2 tsp total: cumin, paprika, turmeric, cinnamon, salt, black pepper (mix to taste)

Tabbouleh Topping:
- 1 cup parsley, finely chopped
- 1 cucumber, diced
- 1 tomato, diced
- 2 tbsp lemon juice
- 1 tbsp olive oil
- Salt & pepper to taste

Instructions

- Preheat oven: 375°F. Grease or line a 12-cup muffin tin.
- Make crust: mix cauliflower, eggs, cheese, olive oil, salt, and pepper. Press half into muffin cups. Bake 7 mins.
- Cook chicken: sauté cubed chicken with spice blend and olive oil until cooked through.
- Assemble & bake: spoon chicken into crusts, top with remaining cauliflower mix. Bake 20–25 mins. Broil 5 mins to crisp.
- Make Tabbouleh: toss parsley, cucumber, tomato, lemon juice, oil, salt, and pepper. Let sit 5–10 mins.
- Serve: top each pie with a spoonful of tabbouleh. Store leftovers in the fridge for up to 4 days.

Scan to watch

Serves 12 mini pies

Prep time 20 min

Cook time 30 min

Quick Tips:
- Want to go vegetarian? Sub the chicken with chickpeas.
- These freeze beautifully—just skip the tabbouleh until serving.

Calories per pie: ~120 | Protein: ~14g | Carbs: ~6g | Fat: ~5g

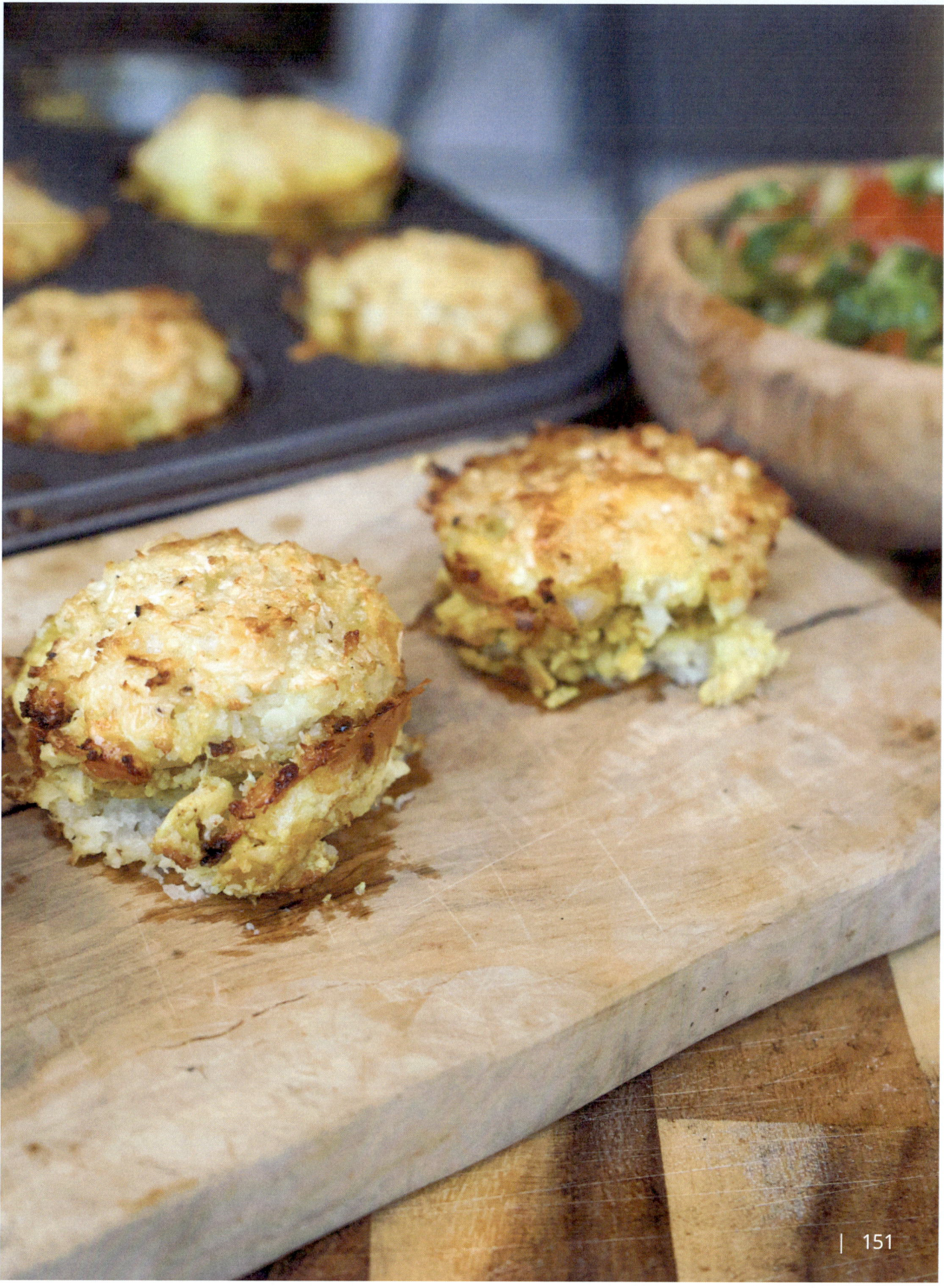

BUTTER CHICKEN WITH CAULI-CABBAGE RICE

This butter chicken keeps the comfort-food vibe but dials up the nutrients. By swapping heavy cream for Greek yogurt and serving it with cauliflower, cabbage, and spinach, you get a high-protein, lower-carb meal that fits into any busy weeknight or meal prep plan.

Ingredients

For the Chicken:
- 2 lb chicken thighs cubed
- 2 tbsp butter, divided
- 1 onion, diced
- 3 cloves garlic, minced
- 2 tbsp garam masala
- 1 tsp each cumin & turmeric
- ½ tsp cinnamon
- Salt & pepper to taste
- 1 can (28 oz) tomato purée or San Marzano tomatoes
- 1 cup Greek yogurt or cottage cheese blended with 1 tbsp lemon juice + splash of milk

For the Veggies:
- 3 cups cauliflower rice
- 3 cups shredded cabbage
- 3 cups baby spinach
- 1 tsp each cumin & garam masala
- Juice of 1 lime

Instructions

- Heat 1 tbsp butter in a large pan. Sauté onion until soft (3–4 min), then stir in garlic and all spices. Cook 1 min until fragrant.
- Add chicken, season with salt and pepper, and brown for a few minutes. Pour in tomato purée, stir, cover, and simmer for 15–20 min.
- Reduce heat and stir in Greek yogurt (or cottage cheese blend). Simmer 5 min more until sauce is creamy and chicken is tender.
- In another pan, melt remaining butter. Sauté cauliflower rice, cabbage, and spinach with cumin, garam masala, and lime juice for ~5 min.
- Spoon butter chicken over veggie rice. Finish with lime juice and cilantro.

Scan to watch

Serves 6

Prep time 10 min

Cook time 20 min

Quick Tips:
- Avoid curdling: add the yogurt (or cottage cheese blend) off heat or over very low heat to keep it creamy, not clumpy.
- Add frozen peas or zucchini noodles for variety.

Calories: ~320 | Protein: ~38g | Carbs: ~18g | Fat: ~10g

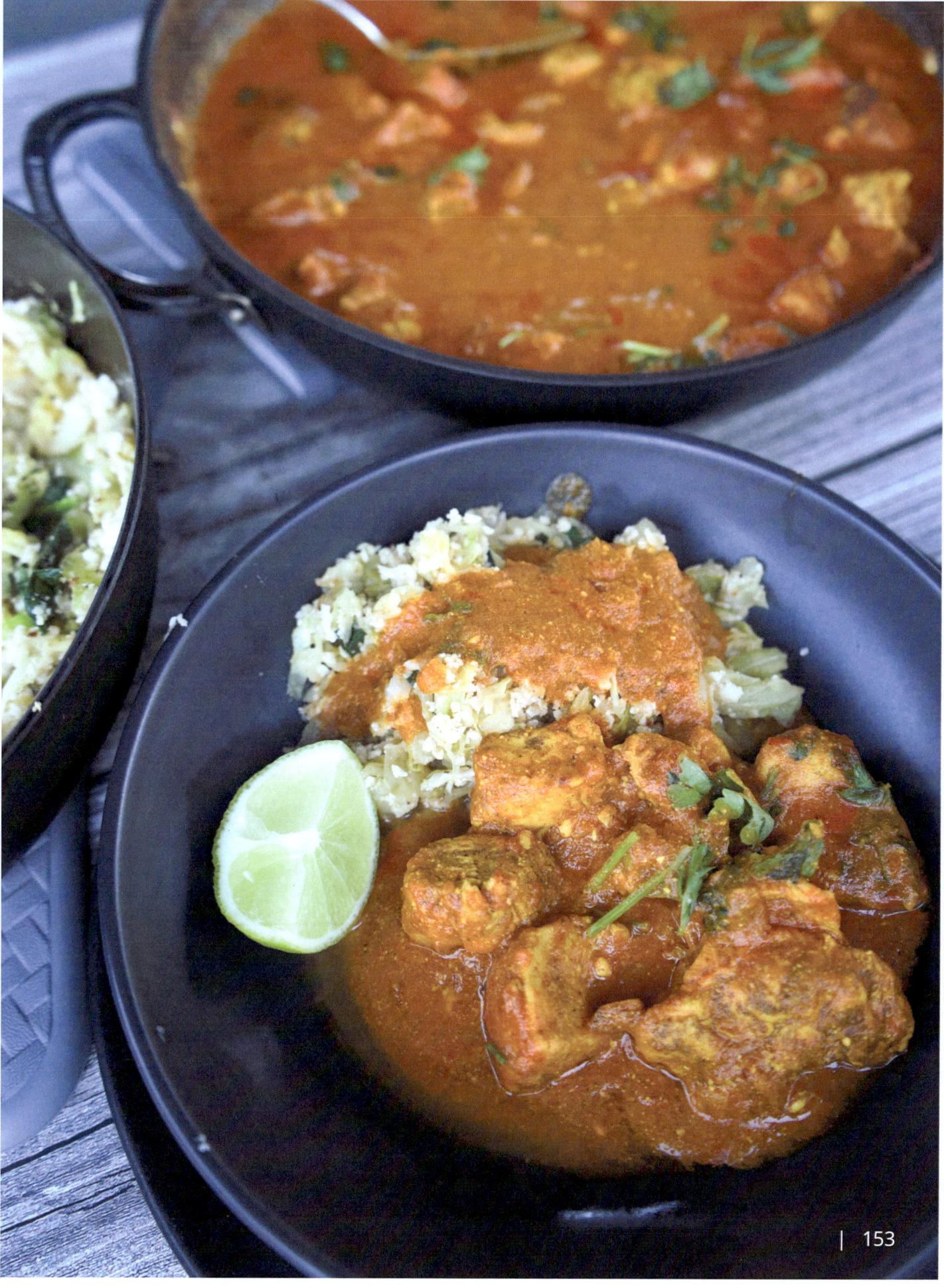

PORK & POTATOES WITH TOMATILLO SAUCE

You don't need a holiday or a dinner party to throw a pork tenderloin in the oven. This version nails the crispy-golden potatoes and adds a citrusy green sauce that's way more exciting than gravy.

Ingredients

Pork Tenderloin:
- 2–3 lb pork tenderloin
- 2–3 tbsp olive oil
- 4 garlic cloves, minced
- 2 sprigs rosemary (or thyme)
- Salt & pepper, to taste

Crispy Potatoes:
- 1 lb baby potatoes, halved
- 2 tbsp olive oil
- 2 garlic cloves, smashed
- ½ tsp smoked paprika
- 1 tbsp fresh rosemary
- Salt & pepper, to taste

Tomatillo-Epazote Sauce:
- 1 lb tomatillos, husked
- 1 small jalapeño
- 1–2 garlic cloves
- Juice of 1 lime
- ½ cup fresh epazote leaves (or substitute with cilantro)
- 1 tbsp honey
- 1 tbsp olive oil
- Salt & pepper to taste

Instructions

- Pat pork dry. Rub with olive oil, garlic, salt, and pepper. Sear in an oven-safe skillet over high heat for 3–4 minutes per side until browned. Add rosemary to the skillet.
- Toss halved potatoes with olive oil, paprika, garlic, rosemary, salt, and pepper. Add to the same skillet around the pork. Roast for 30–40 minutes or until pork hits 145°F internally. Rest the pork under foil for 10 minutes before slicing.
- While the pork roasts, blend tomatillos, jalapeño, garlic, lime juice, epazote, honey, olive oil, salt, and pepper until smooth. Taste and adjust seasoning if needed.
- Slice the pork. Spoon over the tomatillo-epazote sauce and serve with crispy potatoes.

Scan to watch

Serves 4-6

Prep time 10 min

Cook time 50 min

Quick Tips:
- No epazote? Cilantro works just fine—same fresh vibe.
- Double the sauce and save it for grilled chicken or tacos.
- Add a spoon of Greek yogurt or cottage cheese on the side to bump protein

Calories: ~450 | Protein: ~45g | Carbs: ~22g | Fat: ~18g

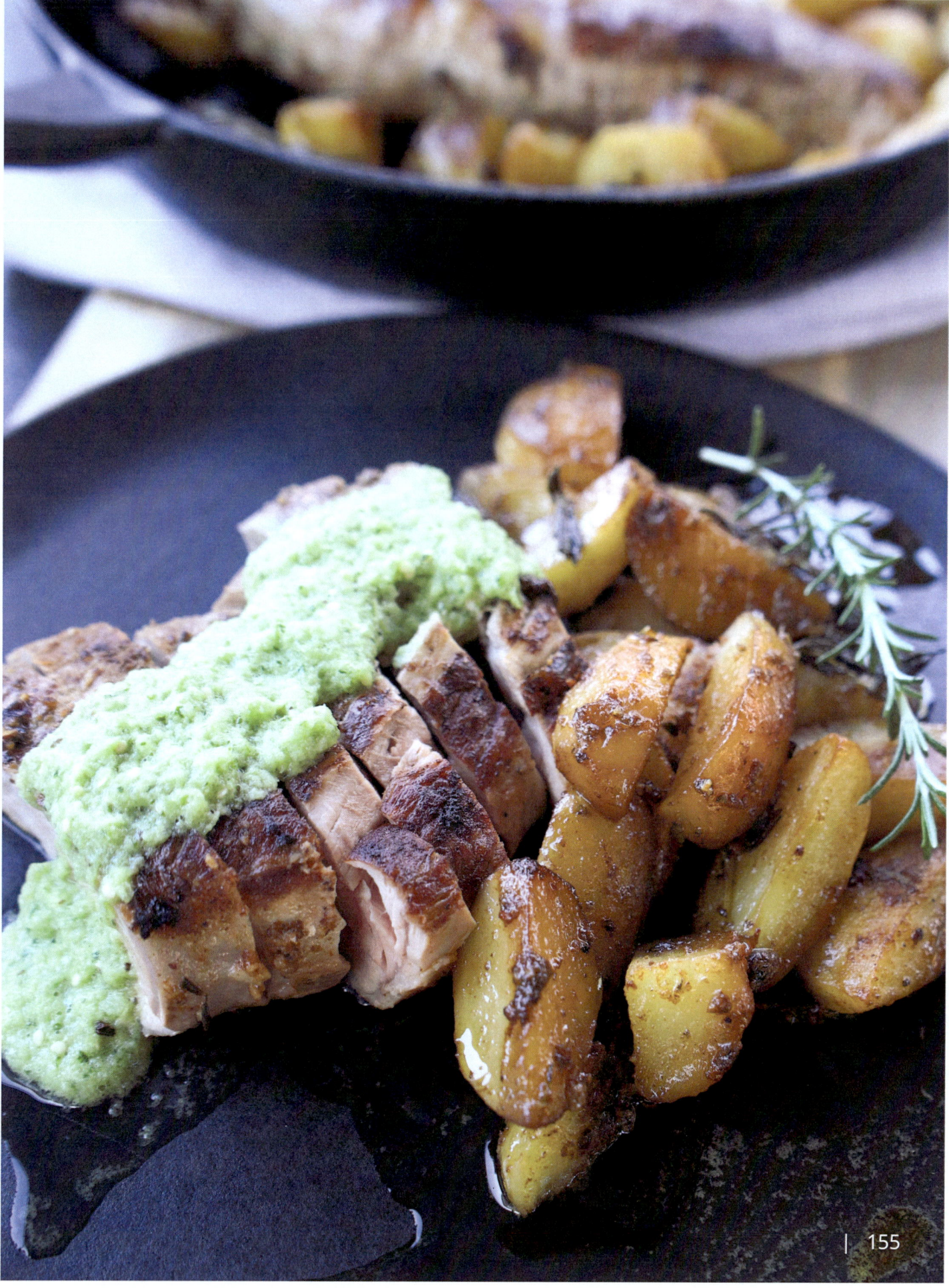

ZUCCHINI BOATS WITH SHRIMP, MARINARA & FETA

When you need something light but still want real flavor, these zucchini boats deliver. Shrimp adds lean protein, the feta gives it tang, and marinara or tomato jam turns this into something borderline gourmet. Fast enough for weeknights, fancy enough for guests.

Ingredients

- **4 medium zucchinis, halved lengthwise**
- **1 lb raw shrimp (about 24 small), peeled & deveined**
- **1 cup marinara sauce (or tomato jam for a sweet-savory twist)**
- **1 cup crumbled feta cheese**
- **2 tbsp olive oil**
- **Salt & pepper to taste**
- **Fresh basil or parsley for garnish**

Instructions

- Preheat oven to 400°F.
- Scoop out zucchini centers with a spoon and arrange cut-side up in a baking dish. Drizzle with olive oil and season with salt and pepper.
- Place 3–4 shrimp in each zucchini half. Spoon marinara or tomato jam over the top and sprinkle generously with feta.
- Bake uncovered for 20–25 minutes, or until shrimp are pink and cooked through and zucchinis are fork-tender.
- Top with fresh basil or parsley. Serve hot. Leftovers reheat surprisingly well, too.

Scan to watch

Serves 4 (8 boats)

Prep time 5 min

Cook time 25 min

Quick Tips:
- Bump the protein: Add ½ cup cottage cheese under the marinara for even more muscle fuel.
- Sweet or savory: Tomato jam brings a caramelized edge, marinara keeps it classic—pick your mood.

Calories: ~200 | Protein: ~18g | Carbs: ~6g | Fat: ~10g

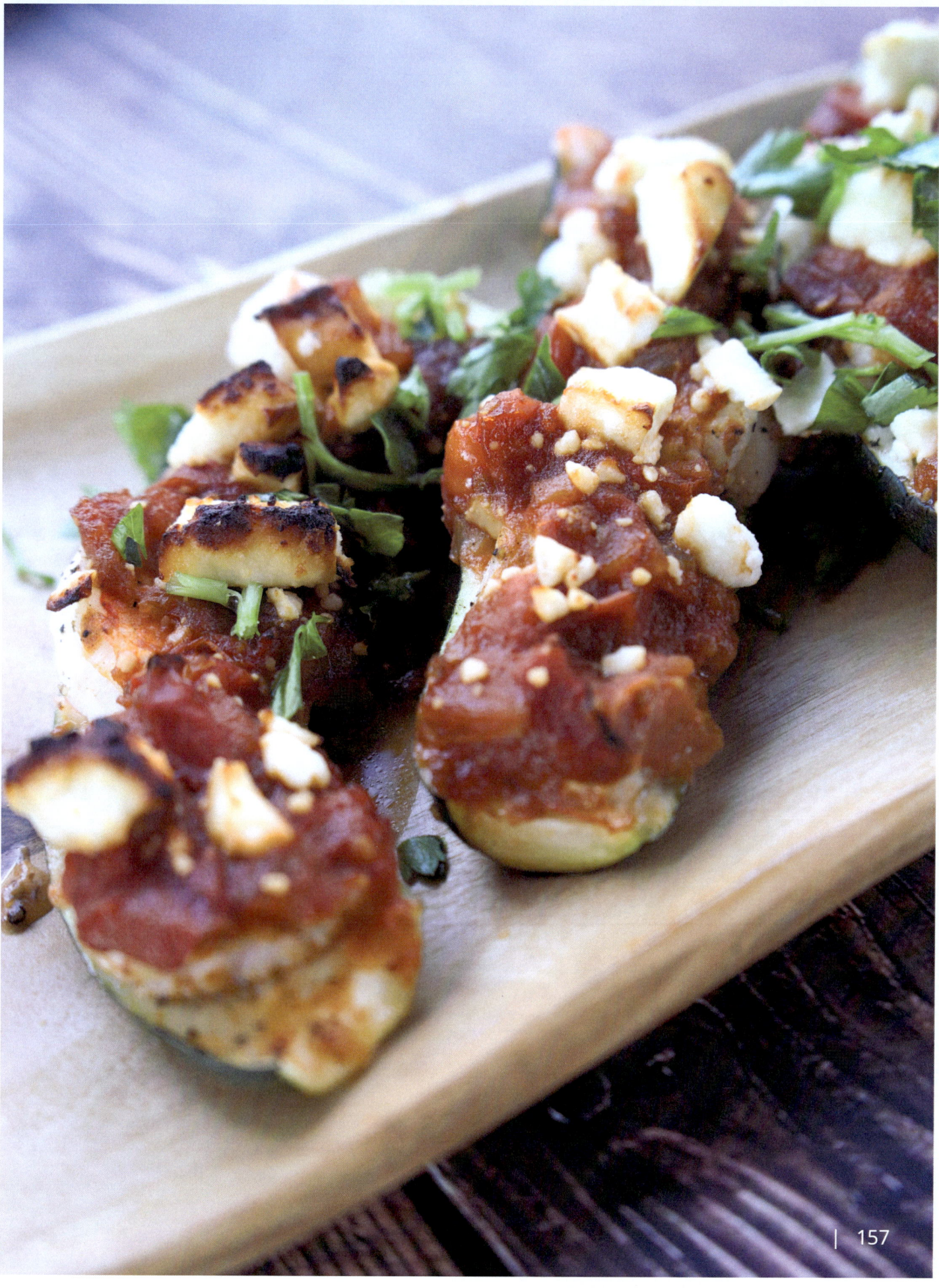

PANANG BEEF CURRY WITH A TWIST

This rich, creamy, coconutty beef curry delivers a peanutty punch and serious comfort in under 30 minutes. Serve it over jasmine rice, or if you're feeling fancy, pile it into a homemade coconut waffle cone.

Ingredients

- **1 lb shaved beef**
- **2 tbsp coconut oil**
- **1 small onion, diced**
- **1 red bell pepper, sliced**
- **3 cloves garlic, minced**
- **1 tbsp fresh ginger, minced**
- **2 tbsp Panang curry paste**
- **1 can (14 oz) coconut milk**
- **½ cup beef broth**
- **2 tbsp peanut butter**
- **1 tbsp soy sauce**
- **1 tbsp fish sauce**
- **1 tbsp brown sugar**
- **1 kaffir lime leaf**
- **1 Thai chili**
- **Thai basil (or cilantro)**
- **Juice of 1 lime**
- **¼ cup crushed peanuts**
- **Cooked jasmine rice or coconut waffle cones for serving**

Instructions

- Heat 1 tbsp coconut oil in a skillet over high heat. Sear beef for 1–2 minutes until just browned. Set aside.
- Add remaining coconut oil. Sauté onion, bell pepper, garlic, and ginger for 2–3 minutes. Stir in curry paste and toast for 30 seconds.
- Stir in coconut milk, broth, peanut butter, soy sauce, fish sauce, and sugar. Add lime leaf, chili and simmer.
- Return beef to the pan. Simmer 2–3 minutes more.
- Stir in Thai basil and lime juice. Remove lime leaf and chili. Serve over rice or in cones. Garnish with crushed peanuts and more basil.
- Coconut Waffle Cones (Makes ~4) Whisk 3 tbsp coconut flour, 2 eggs, 1 tbsp honey, lime zest, pinch of salt, and 3 tbsp coconut milk (adjust for thin batter). Cook on waffle cone maker.

Scan to watch

Serves 4

Prep time 10 min

Cook time 20 min

Quick Tips:
- No waffle maker? Use a pan and make flat wraps instead.
- Choose beef wisely: flank, ribeye, or thin-sliced sirloin work best.
- No Panang paste? Use red curry paste + 1 tsp ground peanuts.

Calories (no rice or cone): 420 | Protein: 25g | Carbs: 10g | Fat: 30g

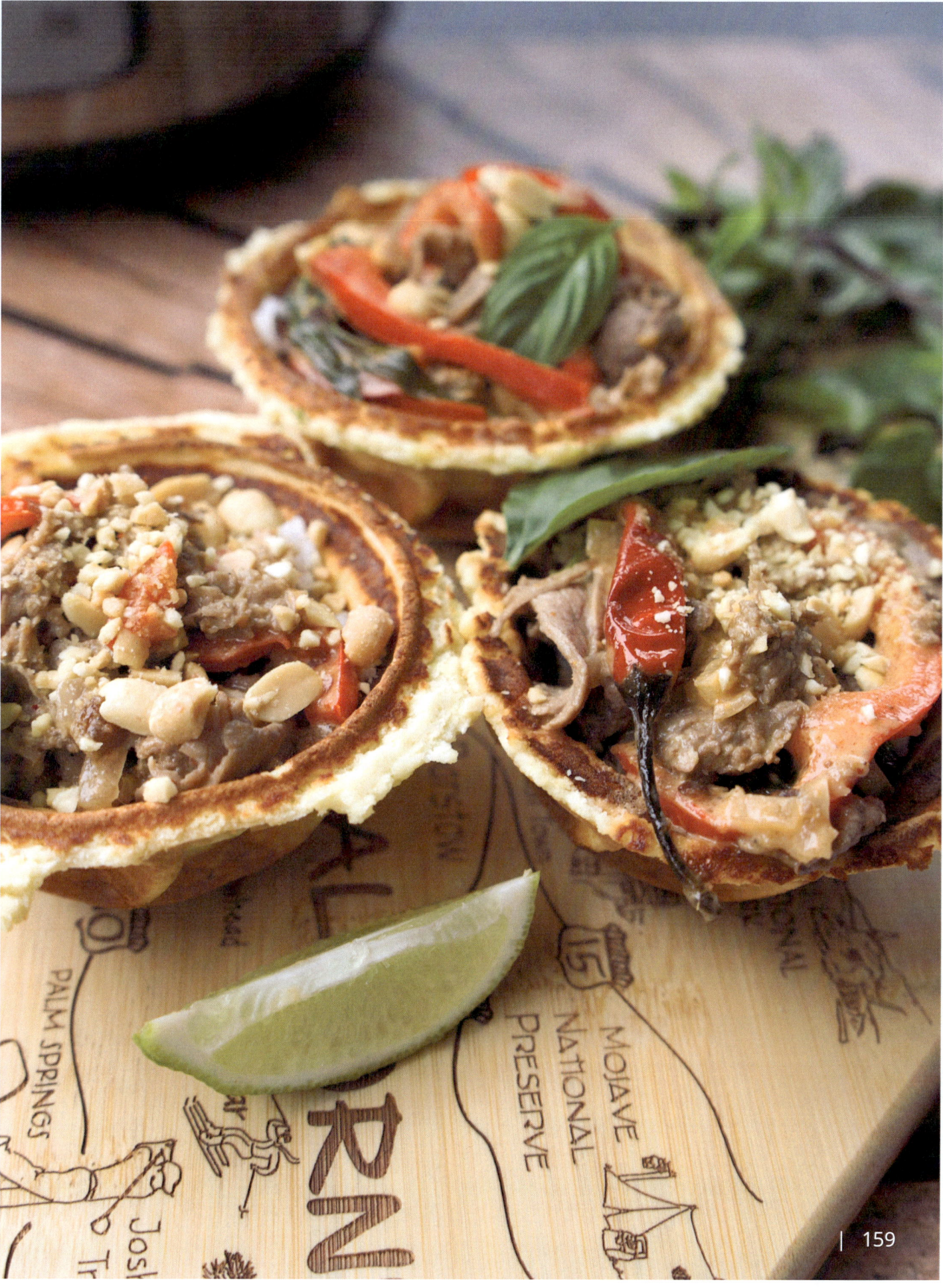

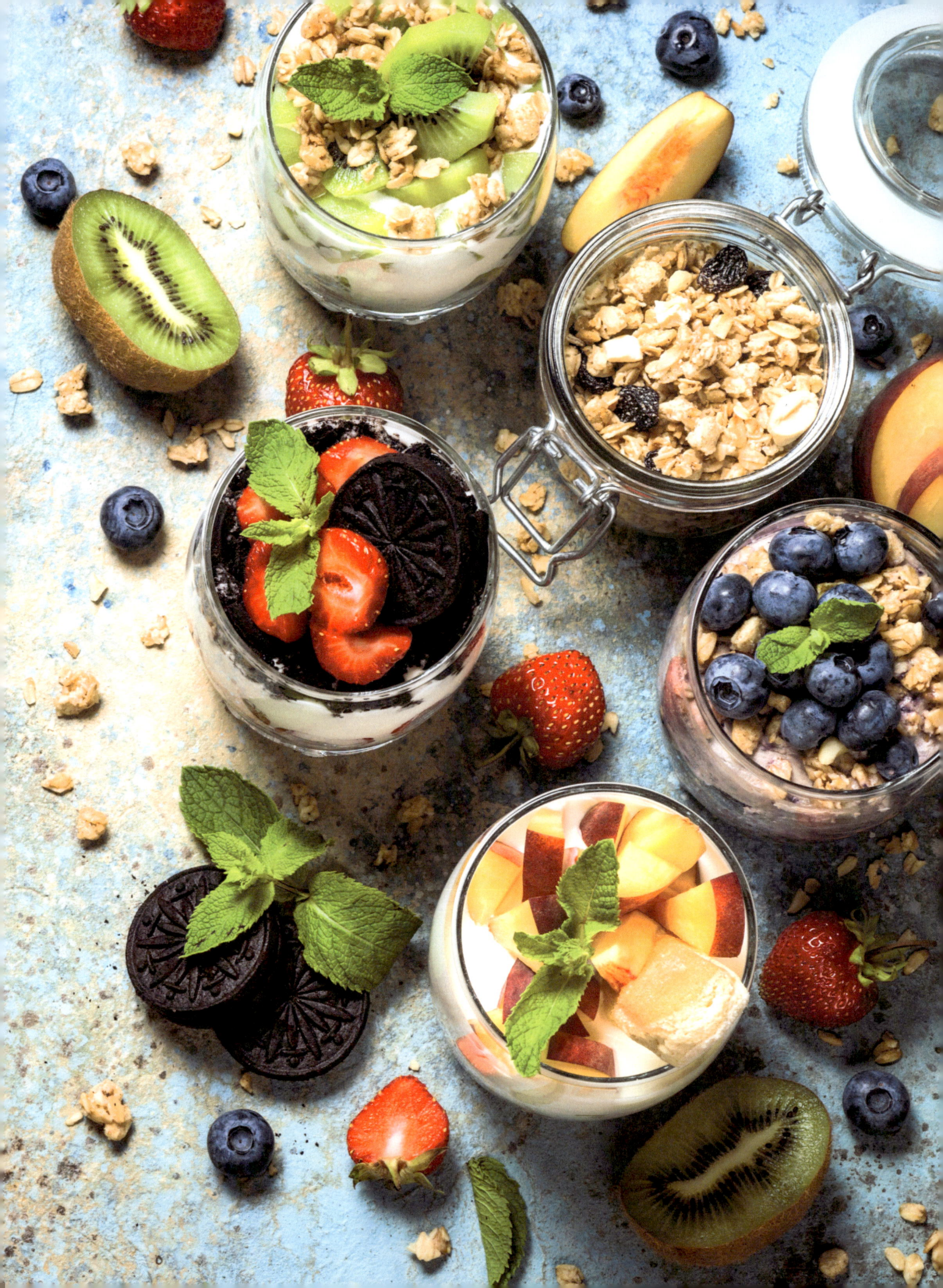

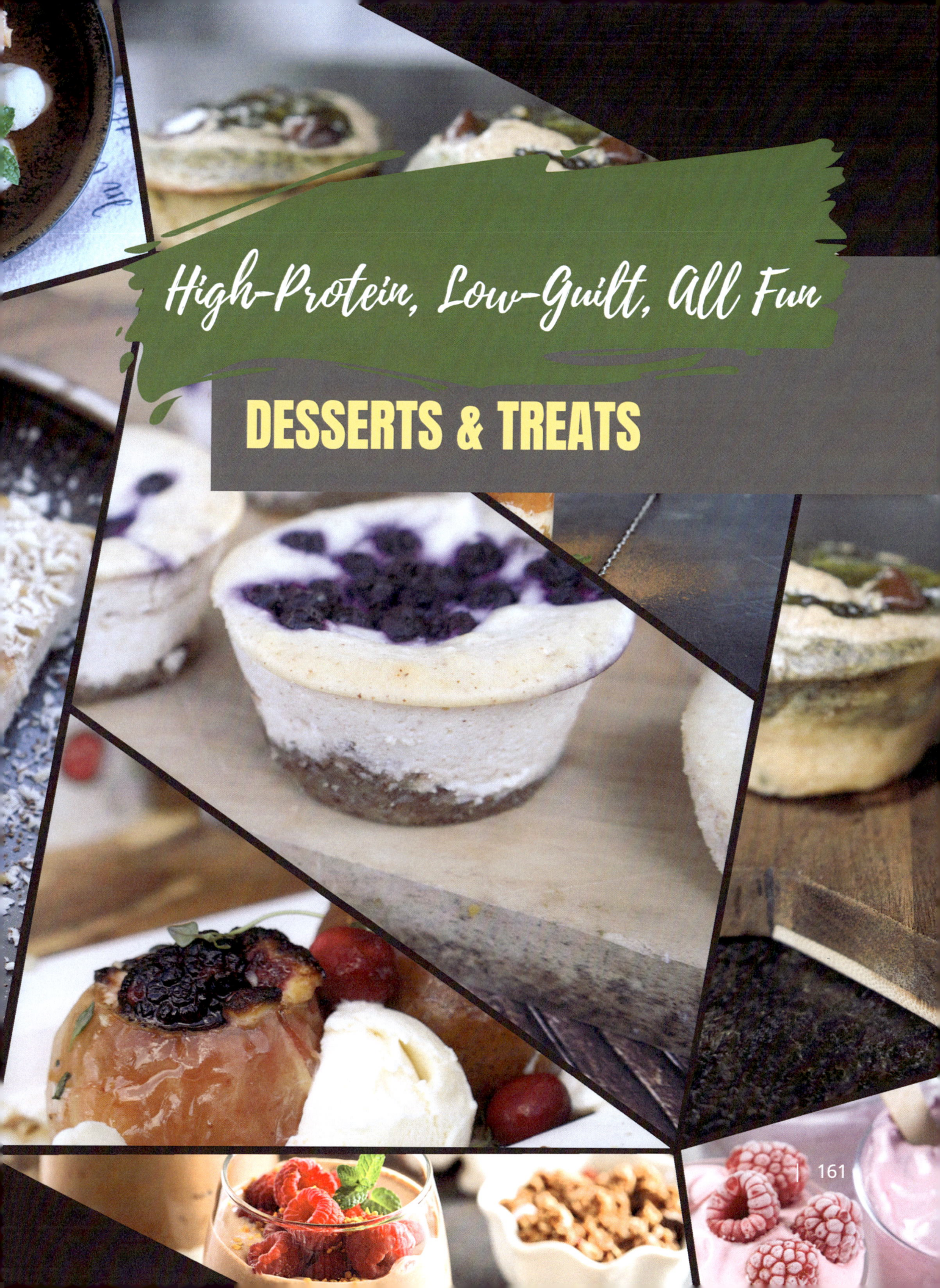

High-Protein, Low-Guilt, All Fun
DESSERTS & TREATS

NUTTY CHEESECAKE BITES

You know that moment post-workout when your biceps are pumped, your legs are jelly, and all you want is a protein bar—but your taste buds are crying for something that doesn't taste like a gym mat? Enter these cheesecake bites. They're creamy, nutty, sweet, and jacked with protein.

Ingredients

Crust:
- 1 cup almond or oat flour
- 1½ tbsp melted coconut oil or butter
- 1 tbsp honey
- 1 tsp vanilla extract

Cheesecake Filling:
- 2 cups blended cottage cheese
- 8 oz cream cheese, softened
- 2 large eggs
- 4 tbsp honey
- 1 tsp vanilla extract
- 2 tbsp lemon juice
- 2½ tbsp almond butter
- 1 tsp baking powder
- Frozen blueberries (for topping)

Instructions

- Bake the bottoms: preheat oven to 325°F. Mix crust ingredients until sandy. Line muffin tin with paper liners, press crust into each, and bake for 5 minutes. Cool slightly.
- Whip the filling: blend cottage cheese smooth. In a large bowl, mix it with cream cheese, eggs, honey, vanilla, lemon juice, almond butter, and baking powder until silky. Pour into muffin cups. Top with blueberries.
- Bake & chill: bake 15–18 min until centers are set but still slightly jiggly. Cool to room temp, then chill at least 2 hrs (or overnight).
- This recipe makes 12 muffin-sized cheesecake bites

Scan to watch

Serves 12

Prep time
15 min

Cook time
20 min

Quick Tips:
- Keeps well in the fridge for a few days. Perfect for meal prep, post-workout snacking, or guilt-free late-night fridge raids.

Calories (per bite): ~150 | Protein: ~10g | Carbs: ~7g | Fat: ~10g

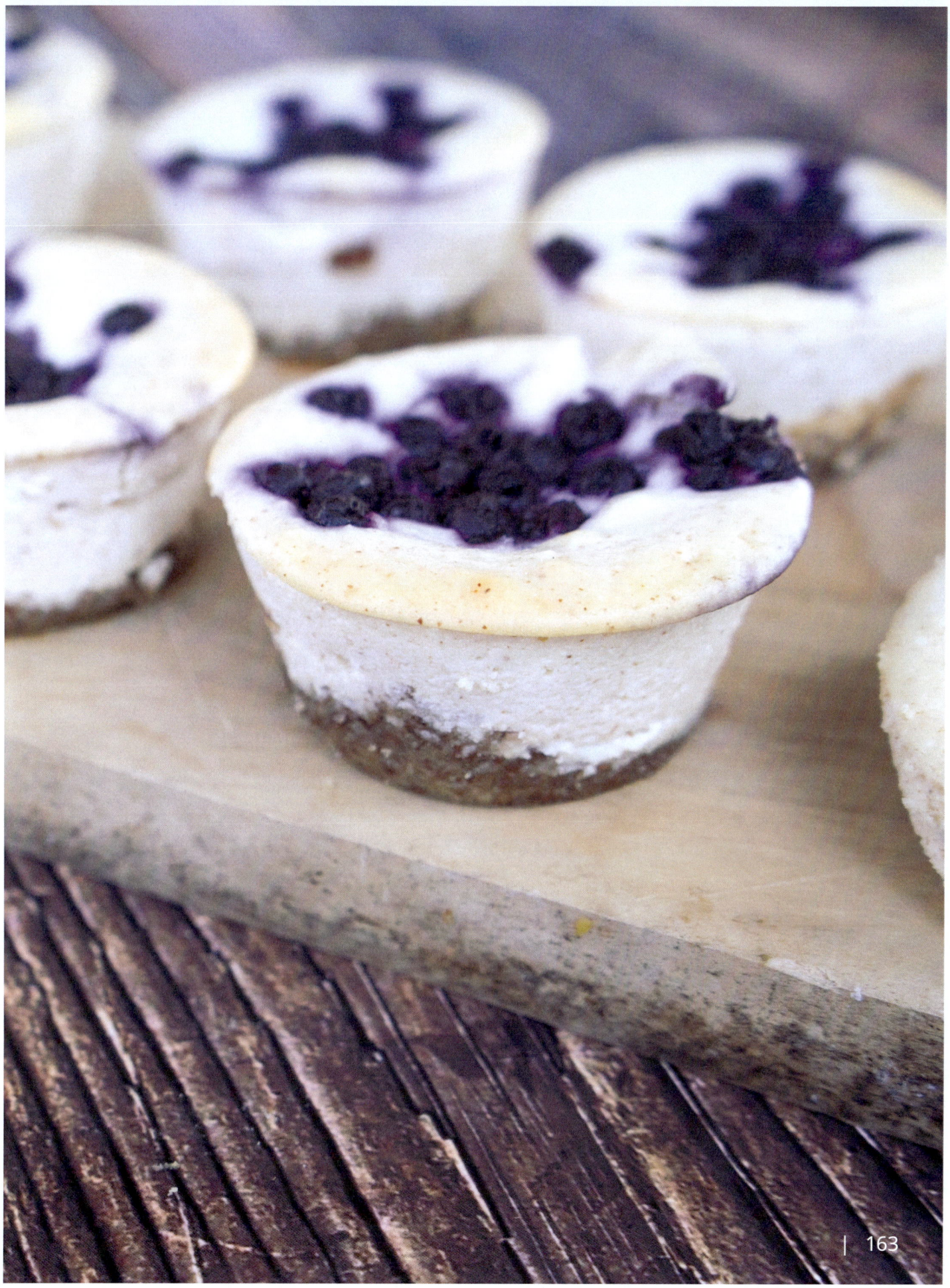

HIGH-PROTEIN HACHIYA PERSIMMON BREAD

So, someone dropped off a truckload of ripe Hachiya persimmons like it was a 19th-century fruit trade. Naturally, I went full mad scientist in the kitchen and Frankensteined my banana bread base into this high-protein, low-carb beauty. No sugar. No regrets. And yes, it has bourbon (optional, but... come on). It's dense, satisfying, and totally snack-worthy for gym rats and brunch snobs alike.

Ingredients

- **7 ripe Hachiya persimmons (pulp only, skin removed)**
- **6 large eggs**
- **1½ cups almond or oat flour**
- **1¼ cups Greek yogurt**
- **1½ tsp baking powder**
- **1½ tsp cinnamon**
- **½ tsp salt**
- **2 tbsp melted coconut oil**
- **1½ tsp vanilla extract**
- **3 tbsp bourbon or whiskey (optional, for flavor flex)**
- **½ cup dried cranberries (unsweetened)**

Instructions

- Scoop out the persimmon pulp and blend until silky smooth.
- Soak dried cranberries in warm water or bourbon for 10 min, then drain.
- Whisk together persimmon pulp, eggs, yogurt, melted coconut oil, vanilla, and bourbon.
- In another bowl, stir together almond flour, baking powder, cinnamon, and salt. Fold dry into wet until you've got a smooth batter.
- Stir in the cranberries. Pour the batter into a greased or parchment-lined loaf pan. Sprinkle more cranberries or pumpkin seeds. Bake at 350°F for 50–55 min, or until a toothpick poked in the center comes out clean.

Scan to watch

Serves 10 slices

Prep time 15 min

Cook time 55 min

Quick Tips:
- Only use super-ripe Hachiyas — soft like jelly. Not ripe? Freeze overnight to speed it up.
- No cranberries? Use chopped dates or raisins.
- Make muffins: Bake in a 12-cup tin at 350°F for 25–30 min.

Calories (per slice): ~190 | Protein: ~10g | Carbs: ~10g | Fat: ~11g

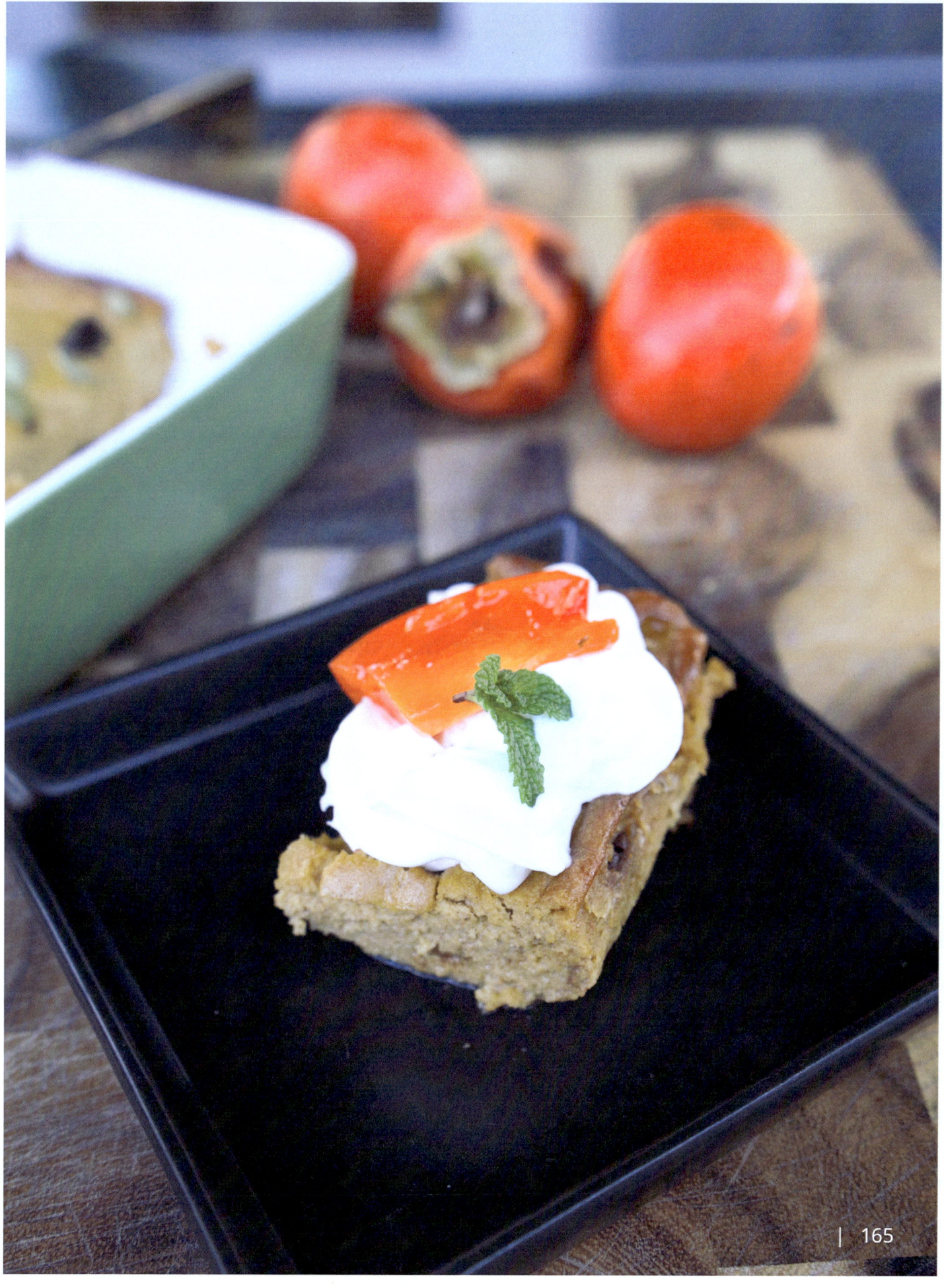

PERSIMMON TIRAMISU TWIST

When life hands you ripe Hachiyas, skip the predictable and go for creamy, dreamy, coffee-soaked glory. It's not a protein bomb—but it's indulgent without the food guilt.

Ingredients

- **3 ripe Hachiya persimmons (pulp only)**
- **1 tbsp cocoa powder**
- **½ cup mascarpone cheese**
- **¼ cup cream cheese**
- **1–2 tbsp condensed milk (to taste)**
- **1 tsp vanilla extract**
- **6 honey graham cookies**
- **1 shot strong brewed coffee**

Instructions

- Make the Persimmon Layer: Blend persimmons with cocoa powder until silky smooth. Set aside.
- Mix the Cream: Whisk mascarpone, cream cheese, condensed milk, and vanilla until smooth. Taste and adjust sweetness.
- Layer It Up: Dip graham cookies quickly in coffee—no soaking! Layer in glasses: cookie → cream → persimmon. Repeat. Finish with cream.
- Chill & Serve: Refrigerate for at least 1 hour. Dust with cocoa powder before serving.

Scan to watch

Serves 2

Prep time
15 min

Chill time
1 hour

Quick Tips:
- Ripe only: persimmons must be soft like pudding. Unripe = bitter.
- Protein boost: stir in a spoonful of Greek yogurt to the cream mix.
- No condensed milk? Use maple syrup + Greek yogurt + a splash of milk.

Calories: ~280 | Protein: ~5g | Carbs: ~35g | Fat: ~14g | Fiber: ~5g

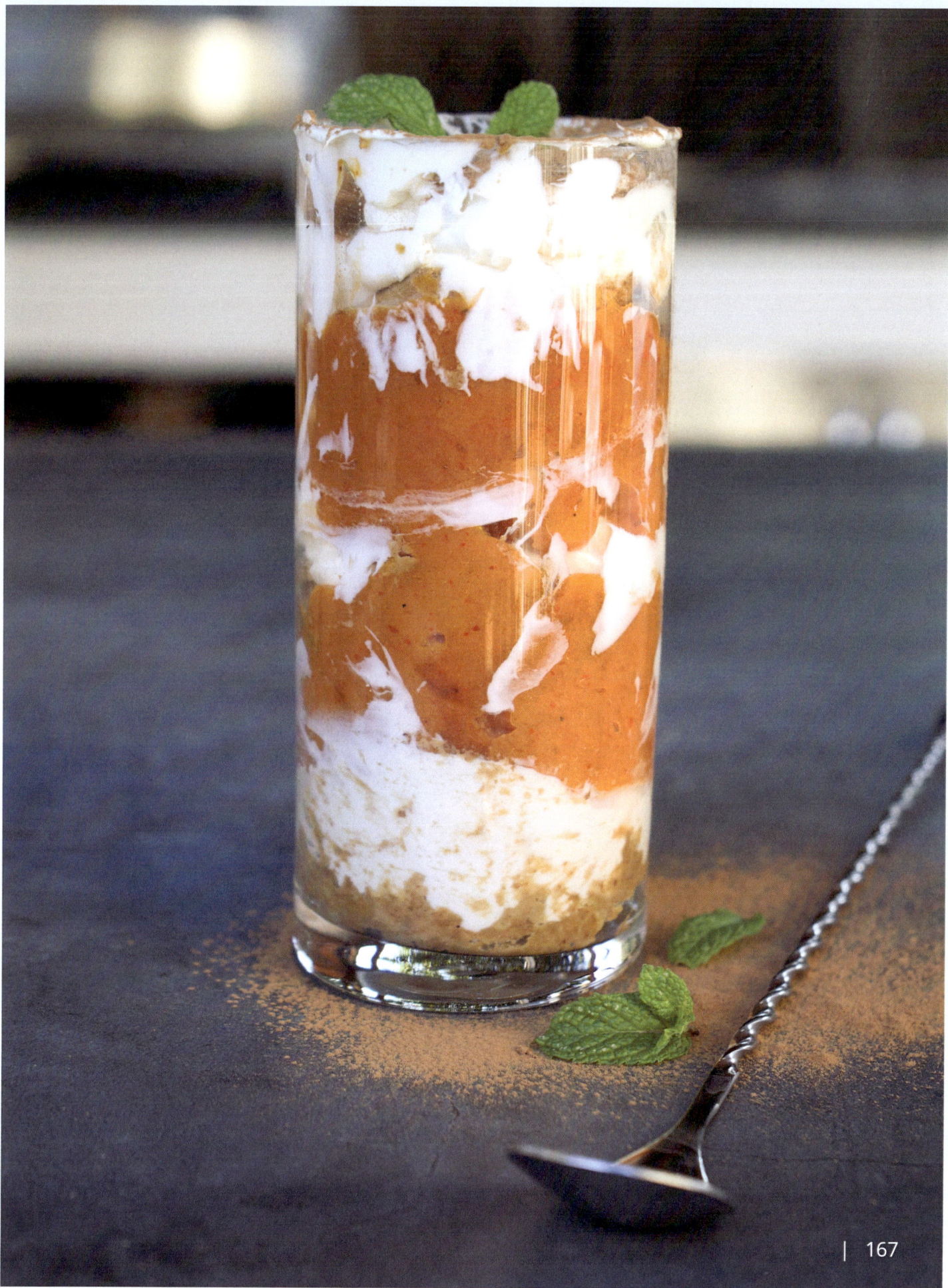

STUFFED APPLES & PEARS WITH FETA & CRANBERRIES

This one's for when you want something light, warm, and dessert-ish without going full sugar bomb. Baked apples or pears get stuffed with cranberries, feta, and berries, then finished with a drizzle of hot honey. Add a splash of Espresso Martini mix if you're feeling like a grown-up. It's simple, satisfying, and flexible enough to suit whatever's in your fridge.

Ingredients

- **4 apples, pears, or apple-pears**
- **¼ cup dried cranberries**
- **4 tbsp feta cheese**
- **4 blackberries (or any berries you love)**
- **1 tbsp extra virgin olive oil**
- **1–2 tbsp hot honey (or regular honey)**
- **¼ cup chopped pecans**
- **Fresh thyme (a few sprigs)**
- **Vanilla ice cream or Greek yogurt (for serving)**
- **Espresso Martini mix (Trader Joe's, optional but fun)**

Instructions

- Slice a thin piece off the top and bottom of each fruit so it stands flat. Carefully core the center without cutting all the way through.
- Add cranberries to the hollow center, followed by 1 tbsp of feta, and cap with a blackberry. Drizzle lightly with olive oil.
- Place stuffed fruits in a baking dish or air fryer. Bake at 375°F for 15–20 minutes, until fruit softens and juices bubble.
- Out of the oven, drizzle with hot honey, sprinkle chopped pecans and thyme, and serve with a scoop of vanilla ice cream or a dollop of Greek yogurt.
- Optional: drizzle with 1–2 tsp of Espresso Martini mix for grown-up flair.

Scan to watch

Serves 4

Prep time 10 min

Chill time 20 min

Quick Tips:
- Feta too salty? Try goat cheese or a mild ricotta.
- No oven? Use the air fryer at 375°F for the same time.
- Want more crunch? Add granola or roasted seeds on top.

Calories: ~200 | Protein: ~3g | Carbs: ~22g | Fat: ~10g
(Without ice cream or martini mix)

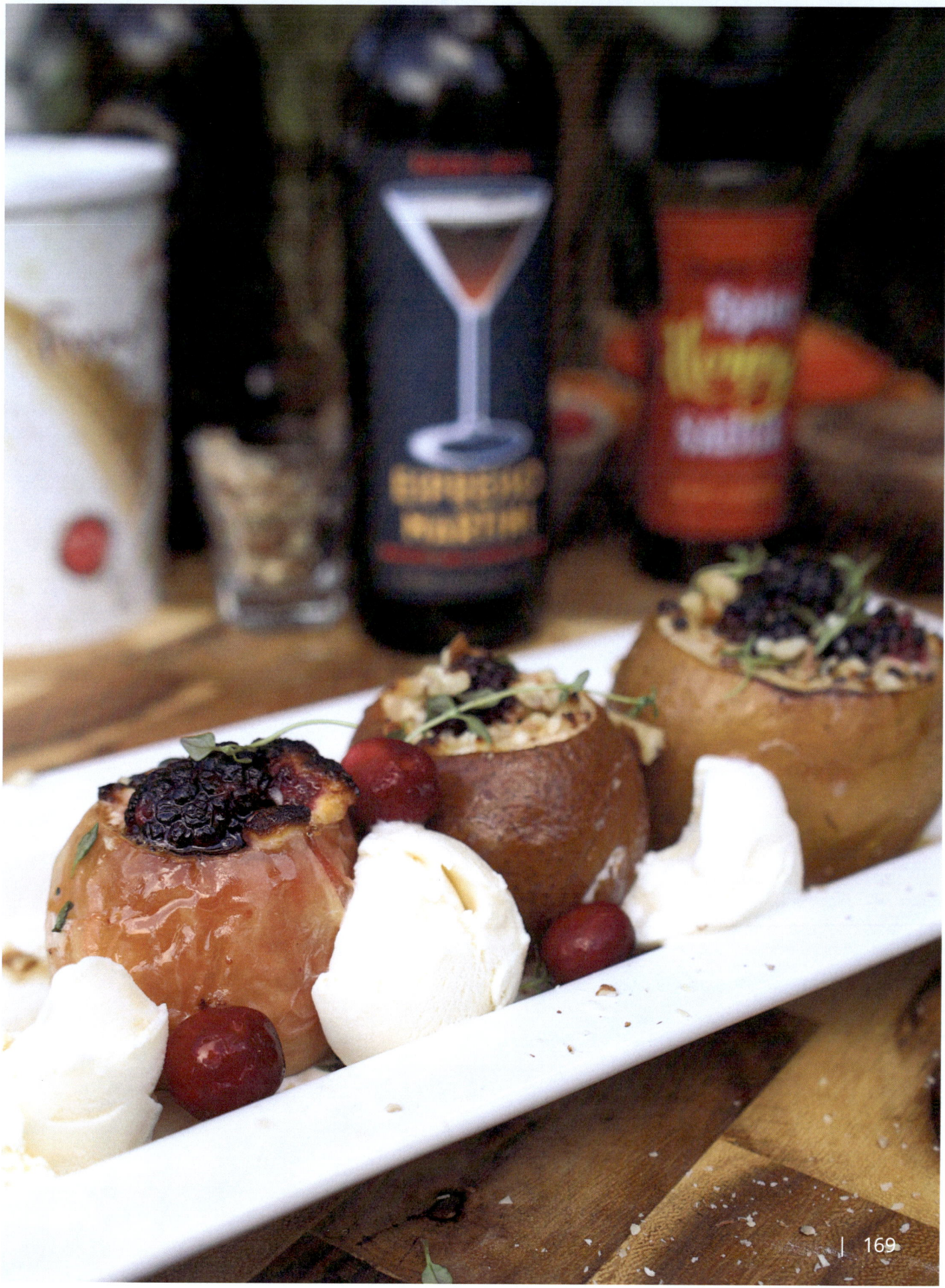

BANANA COCONUT PROTEIN BAKE

Somewhere between a cake and a post-workout reward, this one checks all the boxes: naturally sweet from bananas, tropical from coconut, and packed with protein thanks to egg whites and Greek yogurt. No protein powder needed, and no sugar bomb aftermath. Just slice, chill, and enjoy.

Ingredients

- **2 ripe bananas**
- **1¼ cups coconut or Greek yogurt**
- **¼ cup sugar (adjust to taste or sub with erythritol)**
- **¼ cup grated coconut, divided**
- **1 large egg**
- **½ cup egg whites**

Instructions

- Blend the base: combine bananas, yogurt, sugar, half the grated coconut, egg, and egg whites in a blender. Blend until smooth and creamy.
- Bake it: pour into a greased baking dish (an 8x8" pan works well). Bake at 350°F for about 40 minutes—until golden on top and a toothpick comes out clean.
- Finish & serve: sprinkle the remaining grated coconut on top once baked. Optional: Add a few dark chocolate shavings for flair. Let cool before slicing into 4 servings.

Scan to watch

Serves 4

Prep time
10 min

Chill time
40 min

Quick Tips:
- Use overripe bananas for maximum sweetness.
- Swap sugar for stevia or monk fruit to keep carbs lower.
- Want more protein? Add 1 scoop of unflavored or vanilla whey and bake 5 minutes longer.

Calories: ~210 | Protein: ~17g | Carbs: ~18g | Fat: ~7g

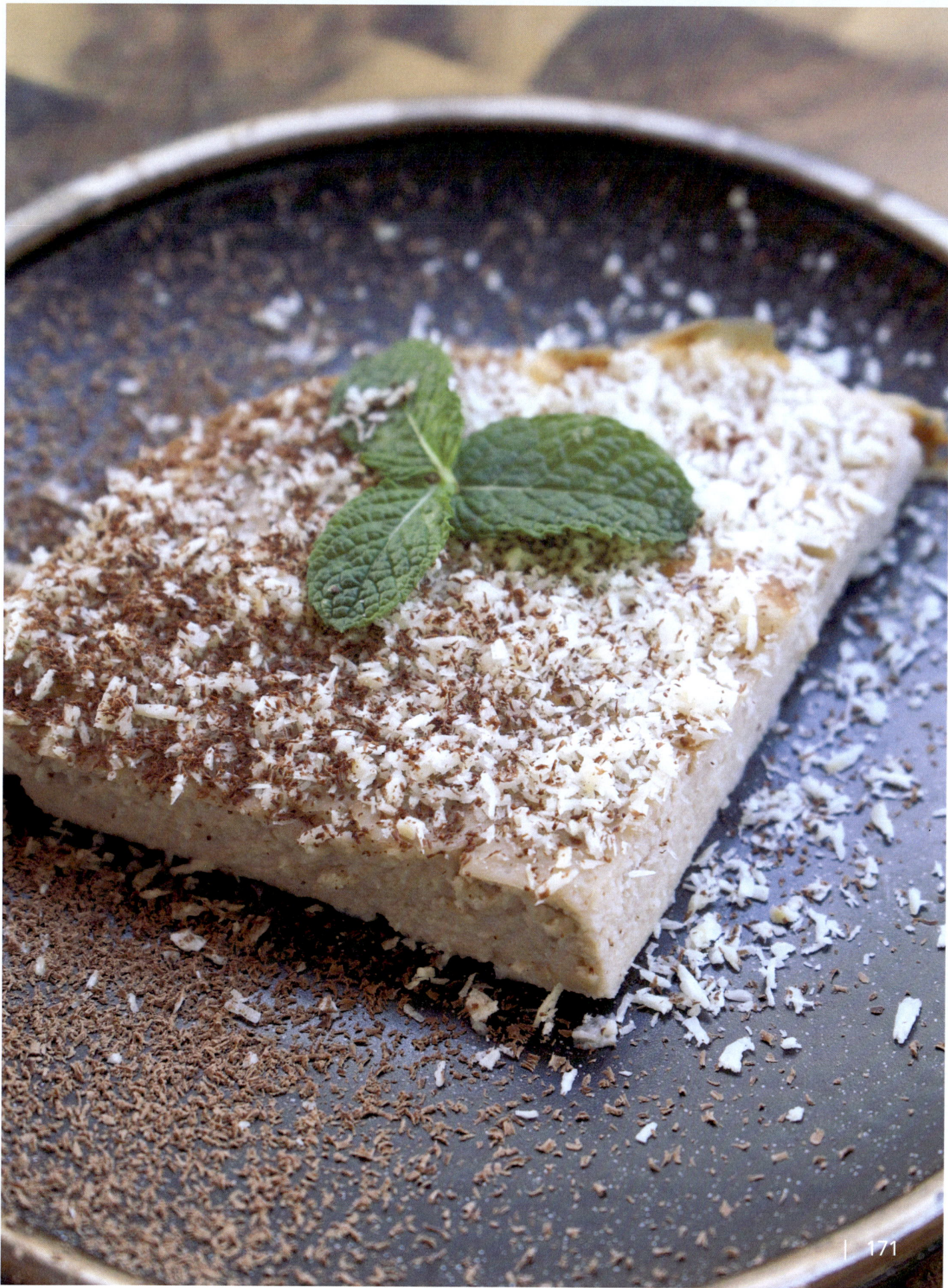

CARAMELIZED PEACHES WITH COTTAGE CHEESE

Juicy peaches meet creamy cottage cheese in this high-protein upgrade to your average snack. Sweet, slightly crispy on the edges, and filled with chocolate chips and chopped nuts—this is what happens when your air fryer decides to get fancy. Dessert? Snack? Post-workout treat? All of the above.

Ingredients

- **4 ripe peaches, halved and pitted**
- **1½ cups regular cottage cheese**
- **2 tbsp honey (optional—skip if your peaches are sweet enough)**
- **3 tbsp mixed nuts, chopped**
- **1 tbsp mini chocolate chips**
- **1 tsp cinnamon**
- **1 tsp vanilla extract**
- **1 tbsp lemon juice**
- **Oil spray for air frying**
- **Fresh mint (optional garnish)**

Instructions

- Preheat & prep: fire up the air fryer to 375°F. Lightly spray the basket with oil.
- Scoop & mix: scoop a bit of flesh out of each peach half, chop it finely, and toss it into a bowl. Add cottage cheese, cinnamon, vanilla, honey, chocolate chips, and chopped nuts. Stir it like you mean it.
- Stuff the peaches: spoon the mixture back into the peach halves. Drizzle with lemon juice for brightness.
- Air fry: place stuffed peaches cut side up in the air fryer. Cook for 15 minutes until the peaches are tender and the tops slightly golden.
- Serve & show off: garnish with fresh mint if you're feeling extra. Serve warm and enjoy immediately.

Scan to watch

Serves 4

Prep time
10 min

Chill time
15 min

Quick Tips:
- Use super ripe peaches for max caramelization.
- No air fryer? Bake at 400°F for 20–25 minutes.
- Boost the protein even more by blending the cottage cheese first for a creamier texture—works great with a scoop of whey added.

Calories: ~270 | Protein: ~19g | Carbs: ~25g | Fat: ~11g

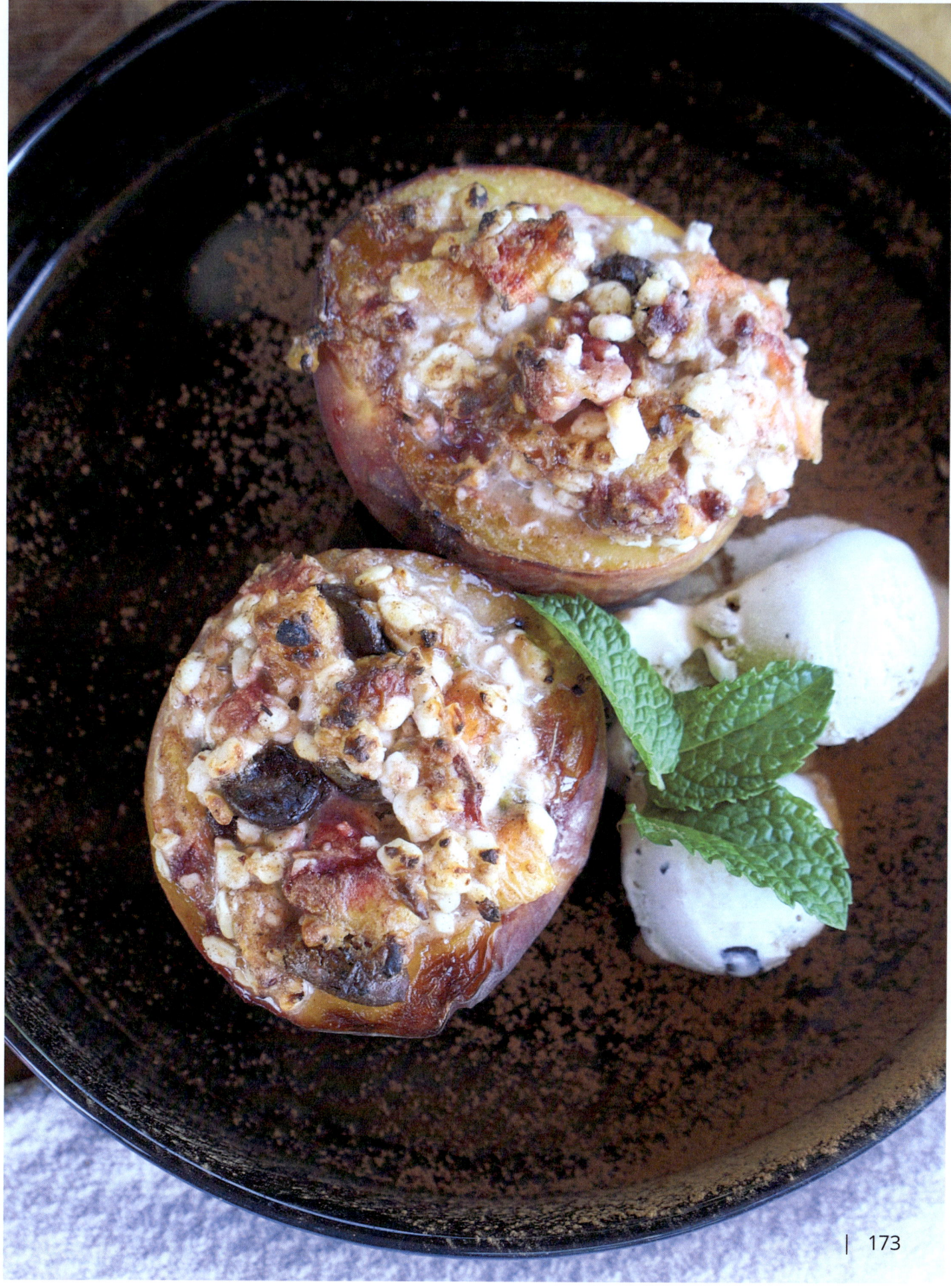

BLUEBERRY CHOCOLATE COTTAGE CHEESE MUFFINS

These muffins are my weekend kitchen side quest with my son. We stir, we spill, we taste-test, and we end up with a dozen fluffy, chocolate-studded, protein-packed muffins that somehow disappear in under 24 hours. If you've got cottage cheese and a blender, you're halfway there.

Ingredients

- **2 cups cottage cheese**
- **4 large eggs**
- **1 cup oat flour**
- **4 tbsp honey**
- **2 tsp vanilla extract (optional)**
- **1 tsp baking powder**
- **½ tsp baking soda (optional)**
- **1 cup blueberries**
- **¼ cup dark chocolate, chopped (optional but excellent)**
- **Pinch of salt**
- **Oil spray (for greasing the muffin tin)**

Instructions

- Preheat your oven to 350°F. In a large bowl or blender, combine cottage cheese, eggs, honey, and vanilla until smooth.
- Fold in oat flour, baking powder, baking soda, and salt. Gently stir in the blueberries and dark chocolate—don't overmix or you'll lose the fluff.
- Lightly spray your muffin tin with oil and divide the batter evenly into 12 muffin cups.
- Bake for 25 minutes or until the tops are golden and a toothpick comes out clean.
- Let cool in the pan before removing. For a sweet crust, sprinkle a pinch of brown sugar on top and broil for 1–2 minutes until caramelized.

Scan to watch

Serves 12 muffins

Prep time 10 min

Chill time 25 min

Quick Tips:
- Want more protein? Add a scoop of vanilla protein powder—just reduce the oat flour slightly.
- Use frozen blueberries if you're out of fresh ones—just don't thaw them.

Calories: ~136 | Protein: ~8.2g | Carbs: ~16g | Fat: ~4.8g

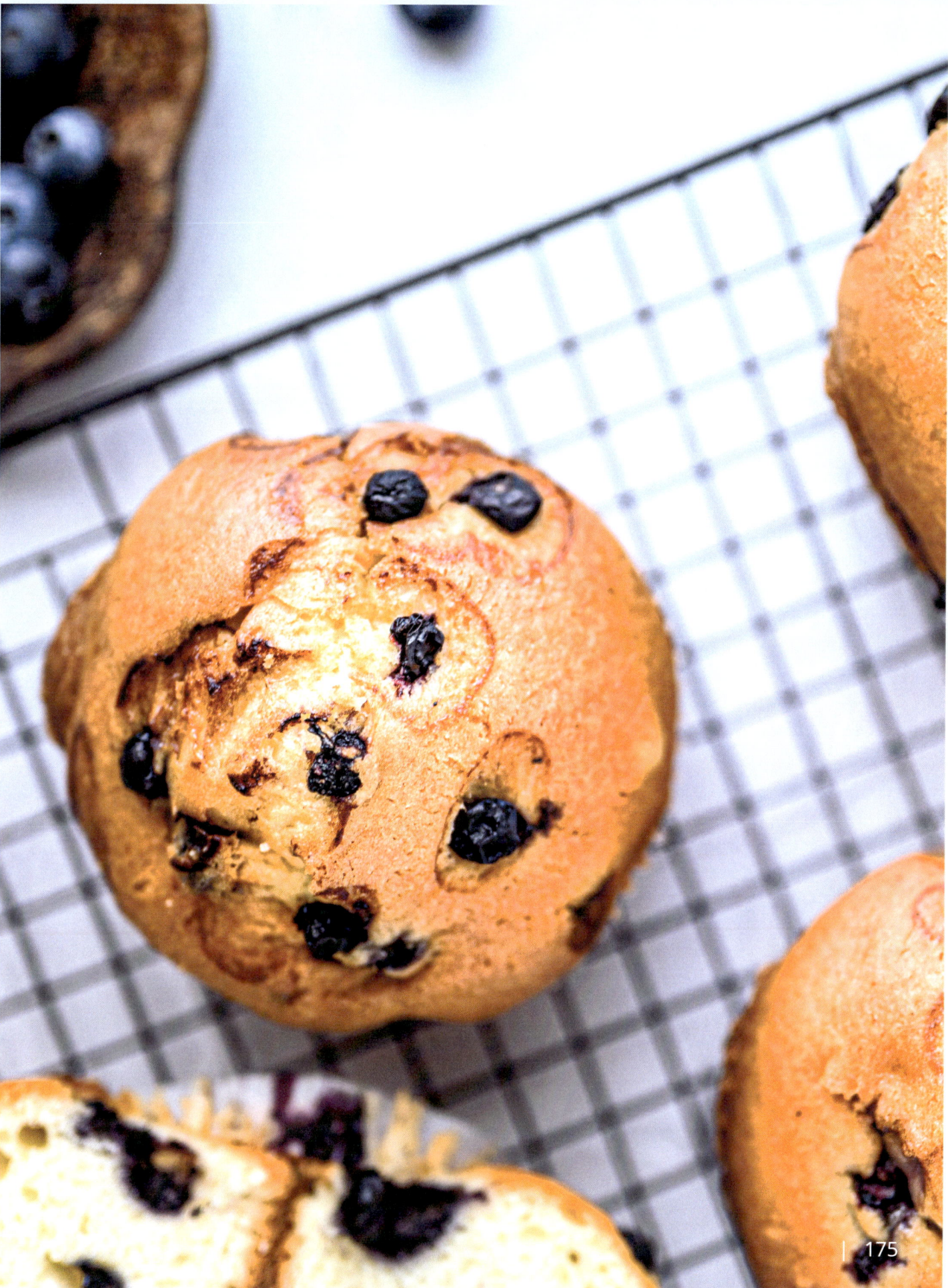

MATCHA ALMOND BUTTER CUPCAKES

These cupcakes are what happens when your post-workout snack and your dessert have a love child. They're soft, subtly sweet, and beautifully green (thanks to matcha, not weird food coloring). Made with cottage cheese, almond butter, and bananas, these guys crush cravings and macros.

Ingredients

For the Cupcakes:
- ⅓ cup almond butter (smooth, unsweetened)
- 4 eggs
- 2 cups cottage cheese
- 4 tbsp honey
- 2 ripe bananas (save ½ of one for layering)
- 1 tsp vanilla extract
- ½ tsp cinnamon
- 1½ cups oat flour
- 3 tbsp matcha powder (culinary grade)
- 1½ tsp baking powder
- ½ tsp salt

For the Topping:
- 2 tbsp almond butter
- 2 tbsp dark chocolate chips
- 1 tbsp honey + ½ tsp matcha powder (whisked together for a quick glaze)

Instructions

- In a bowl, stir together oat flour, baking powder, salt, and cinnamon. Split this mix in half—add matcha powder to one of the halves to create two dry blends.
- In a blender, combine cottage cheese, eggs, honey, vanilla, and 1½ bananas. Blend until smooth and creamy.
- Pour the wet mixture evenly into two bowls. Stir the matcha dry mix into one, and the plain mix into the other.
- Line a muffin tin. Spoon plain batter halfway into each cup, add a banana slice, then top with the matcha batter.
- Drizzle a bit of almond butter on each cupcake. Add a sprinkle of chocolate chips, drizzle the honey-matcha glaze over the top.
- Bake at 350°F for about 25 minutes, or until a toothpick comes out clean.

Scan to watch

Serves 12 cupcakes

Prep time 10 min

Chill time 25 min

Quick Tips:
- For extra protein, replace ½ cup of oat flour with vanilla protein powder—just cut back on the honey by a tablespoon.
- Matcha too earthy? Use only 2 tbsp to start.

Calories: ~145 | Protein: ~10g | Carbs: ~13g | Fat: ~6g

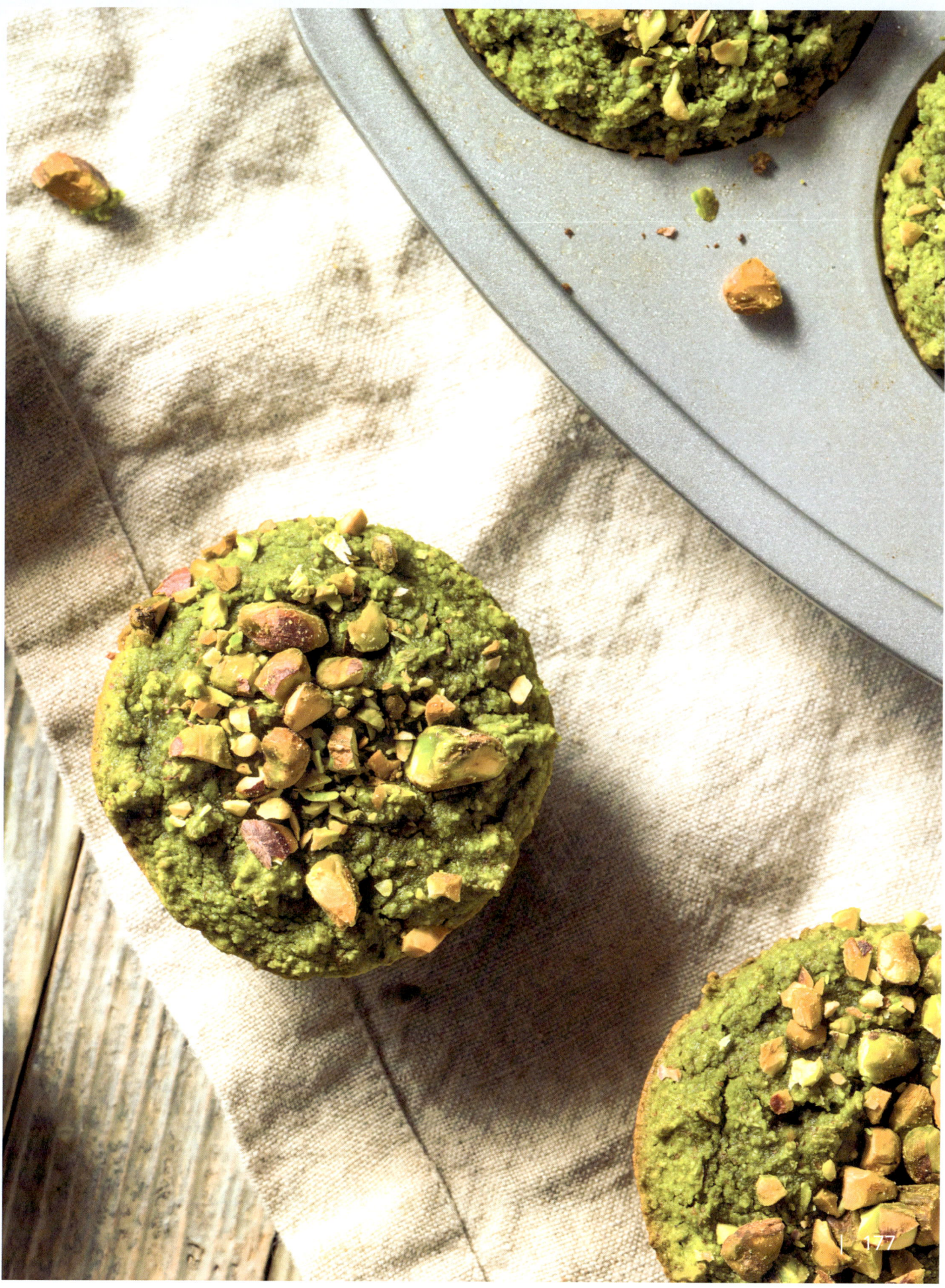

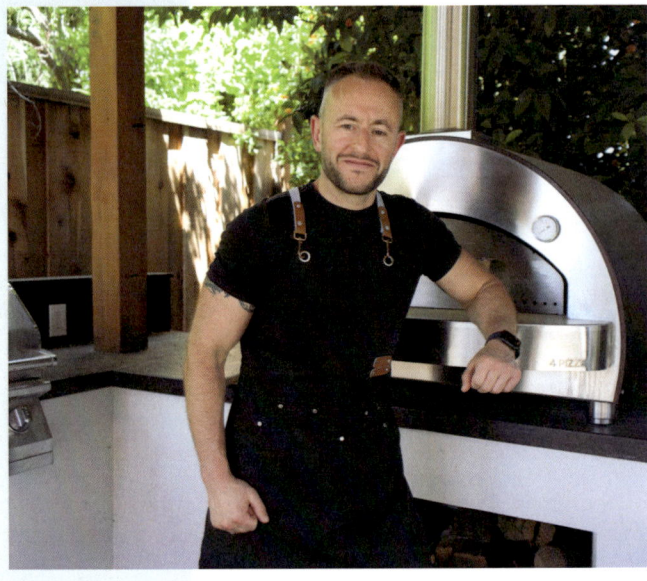

Thank you!

Copyright © 2025 by Ilya Khayn

All rights reserved. No part of this publication may be reproduced, distributed, or transmitted in any form or by any means—whether photocopying, recording, or other electronic or mechanical methods—without the prior written permission of the author, except in the case of brief quotations used in reviews, articles, or social media shoutouts (tag me, obviously).

Book Title: Quick Fit Kitchen, Low-Carb, High-Protein Meals with International Flavor
Author: Ilya Khayn
First Edition, 2025
ISBN: 979-8-9992523-0-2

All content, photography, and design were created by the author unless otherwise noted. Select visual elements and images were sourced and licensed from Canva.com in accordance with Canva's Content License Agreement.

Brand names and logos appearing in photographs or recipes are the property of their respective owners. Their appearance in this book is purely incidental and does not imply endorsement or sponsorship unless explicitly stated.

Select quotations from Julia Child are used under fair use for educational and inspirational purposes. Julia Child is a registered trademark of The Julia Child Foundation for Gastronomy and the Culinary Arts. This book is not affiliated with or endorsed by the Foundation.

This book is intended for informational and entertainment purposes only. The recipes and nutrition information reflect the author's experience as a fitness and food creator. Always consult a qualified professional for medical, fitness, or dietary advice tailored to your needs—or at the very least, use common sense in the kitchen.

Published by Ilya Khayn
@inthekitchenwithilya

Stay in touch!

"This is my invariable advice to people: Learn how to cook—try new recipes, learn from your mistakes, be fearless, and above all, have fun!"
— Julia Child

www.ingramcontent.com/pod-product-compliance
Lightning Source LLC
Chambersburg PA
CBRC090058100526
44582CB00013B/182